A Death on
Diamond Mountain

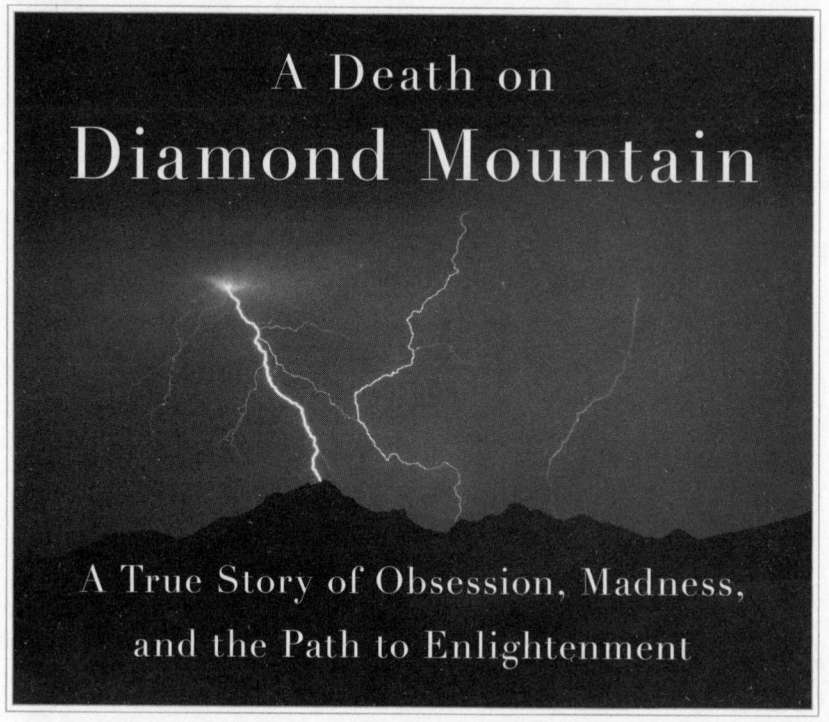

A Death on
Diamond Mountain

A True Story of Obsession, Madness,
and the Path to Enlightenment

SCOTT CARNEY

GOTHAM BOOKS

GOTHAM BOOKS
Published by the Penguin Group
Penguin Group (USA) LLC
375 Hudson Street
New York, New York 10014

USA | Canada | UK | Ireland | Australia | New Zealand | India | South Africa | China
penguin.com
A Penguin Random House Company

Title page photo courtesy of James BO Insogna/Shutterstock.com.

LIBRARY OF CONGRESS CATALOGING-IN-PUBLICATION DATA
has been applied for.

ISBN 978-1-592-40861-0

Printed in the United States of America
1   3   5   7   9   10   8   6   4   2

Set in Dante
DESIGNED BY KATY RIEGEL

For Laura and Allison,

my sisters

Contents

The mind is everything; what you think, you become.
—A COMMON MISQUOTE OF THE BUDDHA

The universe is made of stories, not of atoms.
—MURIEL RUKEYSER

Author's Note

How MUCH SHOULD someone strive to know their own soul?

It is a question I have struggled with for the better part of a decade after an incident that taught me that intensive meditation has the potential to unleash unexpected consequences. From 1998 to 2006, I spent about three years bumping around India, Tibet, and Nepal, first as a student on an abroad program learning about Indian and Tibetan folklore, and later in backpacker hostels on the beaches of Goa and the mountain valleys of Kathmandu. Later, I dropped out of a PhD program in anthropology to lead an abroad program for American students that advertised in glossy brochures with the catchy title "India: From Brahma to Buddha." I was excited to help guide young people on their journeys in a foreign land.

The highlight of the program was a ten-day silent meditation retreat in the rustic town of Bodh Gaya, the spot where Buddha achieved enlightenment while sitting under a fig tree almost three millennia ago. We studied an introductory program known in Tibetan as *lamrim* to learn about the karmic cycle of death and rebirth and to cultivate an attitude of compassion for all living things. We were told that this could lead the way to happiness in this life—and perhaps enlightenment in our next.

I began studying Tibetan Buddhism on my first trip to Asia and it had helped me find my own answers to some of life's big questions. Its focus on mortality made me realize that no matter what we believe happens after death, our time on this earth is precious. Buddhists reflect openly on death and teach that although all life ends in tragedy, the way we use our lives does not have to be meaningless. Every moment has value and meditation is one way to capture life's fleetingness.

The first seven days of the retreat consisted mainly of breathing exercises and lectures on the Tibetan worldview. On the eighth day, the experience turned dark. The Swiss-German nun who was our instructor told us to imagine that we were decaying corpses and that the bodies of everyone we knew were bags of human shit. The exercise, which is meant to help the students develop psychic tools to use when they eventually face their own death, might sound extreme, but Tibetan meditation can get even more far-out: A practice known as *chöd* involves meditating over actual decaying corpses in a graveyard.

When the meditations were over, I had a conversation with one of my students—a whip-smart twenty-one-year-old Southern belle named Emily O'Conner (not her real name)—about her experiences.* She said it was the most profoundly moving experience of her life and that "maybe more silence would have been better."

That night, while the other students chatted enthusiastically in the meditation room, she climbed to the roof of one of the dormitories, wrapped a *khadi* scarf around her face, and jumped. A student on his way to bed found her facedown on the pavement. According to the coroner's report, she had died on impact.

I was charged with returning her remains to America. Somewhere along the way, the Indian police gave me her journal. On the eighth day of the retreat, she'd written in flowery, well-constructed

---

*At various points in this book I have changed the names and some details of sources in order to protect their identities.

cursive, "Contemplating my own death is the key." Then, a few paragraphs later, "I'm scared that I will have this realization and go crazy." One of the last things Emily wrote, in the same steady hand, was "I am a Bodhisattva"—an enlightened being that Tibetans aspire to become. She believed she was well along the road to transcendence.

There are many explanations for why Emily, my student, decided to take her own life. Maybe she had misunderstood the meaning of "enlightenment." Maybe she had underlying mental instabilities that just happened to manifest themselves during intensive meditation. For all I knew, she *was* a Bodhisattva and continuing on her journey in another realm. However, here on earth I worried that enlightenment might not be all that it promised.

The experience changed my life, turning me toward a career as an investigative journalist. As I recounted in my book *The Red Market: On the Trail of the World's Organ Brokers, Bone Thieves, Blood Farmers, and Child Traffickers*, my fight to preserve her body with ice and embalming fluid against the inevitability of decay made me consider the subtle line that separates the flesh of a corpse from that of a living person. Without that mysterious animating force that some people might call a soul, our bodies are little more than meat. Out of a living context, that meat is a sort of commodity in the eyes of the world. For the next five or six years, I followed that realization to what, for me, were its logical conclusions. I became a journalist and explored the growing, illegal markets for bodies and body parts.

Even as I pursued criminals across international lines, I often drifted back to the question of why my student took her life. For me, it was more difficult to understand how a technique that was supposed to make someone a more compassionate person could have such a tragic result.

The death of a second meditator, Ian Thorson, this time in the mountains of Arizona, made me suspect that there was an unspoken mystery at the heart of these transformational techniques. There was no doubt that his death and Emily's were rare events—perhaps even within the statistical norms for suicide or murder in a given population. But there were eerie similarities.

Was there something in the teachings that drives some people to madness? Could silence itself be damaging? Or was it something about the way Westerners think about Eastern spirituality that makes us particularly susceptible to grandiose expectations? When not tempered, perhaps that search for something greater than ourselves is enough to push some people past a breaking point.

I began my investigation expecting to uncover a hidden dark side of meditation and yoga that gets swept under the rug. People who adhere to Eastern teachings might be inclined to explain away negative events as the fault of the individual and not of the techniques. To some degree, that *is* what I found. But I also found something stranger. Maybe instead of thinking of spiritual practices as something in and of themselves good or bad, it is more fruitful to think of them as potentially powerful.

Whatever gets unlocked in the meditation chamber, a prayer hall, or a yoga studio is certainly deeply personal, physical, psychological, and subject to the grand sweep of history. There is also something about it that is transcendent, and essential to who we are as humans.

Prologue

The Cave

CHRISTIE MCNALLY'S HAIR hung down in greasy unwashed cords as she scanned the retreat valley with her tired brown eyes. The searing yellow flashlight beams hadn't cut across the tract for at least a week, but that didn't mean their pursuit was over. A month earlier, devotees had bowed at her feet and laid garlands of flowers on her throne. Now guards patrolled the property line, wary of any attempt she might make to reassert control of her flock. Her white robes, long since soiled, were packed away in one of the watertight Rubbermaid tubs that they'd stashed beneath the cave they now occupied.

There were still a few of their loyal Buddhist followers out there somewhere. She'd written a message to them in a bubbly girlish scrawl. Her struggle had a place in the grand sweep of history of the landscape. They'd been expelled from their own slice of Eden and hounded so that she and her husband, Ian Thorson, had "started to feel this terrible sense of being hunted, like a wild rabbit, or perhaps like an Apache of long ago." It was an apt metaphor. A hundred and fifty years earlier, Indians armed with rifles and stolen ammunition squatted on a ridge not far from here. They watched the valley as Union soldiers refreshed their canteens at Bear Spring and waited for the perfect moment to strike. As the soldiers quenched their thirst, the reports of Apache rifles echoed off the canyon walls. Two bullets found their mark. The privates bled out within minutes; their blue uniforms turned purple and the ground soaked up their blood as greedily as it did their spilled canteens. The lieutenant survived to record their passing in a report to his commanding officer at Fort Bowie, whose low adobe walls stood only a quarter mile away.

The murders were just another step in the tit-for-tat violence that culminated in seventy-five years of barbarism known by the victors as the Indian Wars. Vestiges of that violence remained when McNally helped raise money to buy the valley in 2008 and rechristen it Diamond Mountain. Bear Spring silted over and stopped flowing only a few months after the Buddhists arrived. Some locals thought it was a sign.

When they moved here, McNally and Thorson saw the cave as a spiritual refuge in the tradition of the great Himalayan masters. Their plan was as elegant as it was treacherous: They would occupy the cave until they achieved enlightenment. They didn't expect that they might die trying.

Ian Thorson was thin now. Too thin, really. The knife wounds in his sides and shoulders had healed cleanly, but now a fresh bruise swept across his forehead. He'd been delirious for some time, and in his frustration he'd smashed his head with a piece of hardened plastic. It wasn't his fault that the situation didn't make sense anymore. She worried about him hurting himself further. Then again, he was so close to greatness.

McNally knew that when he looked up from the mattress they'd hauled up to their mountain cave, he wouldn't see the guileless face of the girl who grew up outside of Los Angeles: the product of an affair between her father and his secretary. Nor would he identify the outline of the woman with whom he'd helped build Diamond Mountain University into a major site for Tibetan Buddhist meditation. It was not the woman with whom he'd spent countless hours perfecting the intricate postures of couples yoga, where they would use each other's weight to push their bodies into impossible configurations. She certainly wasn't the ex-wife of his first guru and spiritual teacher, Geshe Michael Roach, who was still jealously stewing over their controversial split. No. When he gazed out of the dimming aperture of the cave, he would see an angel made of clear white light. Christie McNally was his lover and his lama, the enlightened being who had seen the nature of emptiness directly, who had married him and taken his tortured soul from a base understanding of the world to the cusp of his own transformation.

She was also his only hope for making it out of here alive.

Even if he could stand, the cave was barely tall enough for Thorson to be on his feet without craning his six-foot frame. During daytime, a small sliver of light filtered in through a hole in the roof where the rocks formed a cleft. It was stuffed with all the things they had thought they would need to survive a long haul. There were bags of basmati rice, bolts of clothing and cold-weather gear, flashlights and jars of Italian seasoning. A small ritual instrument hung from a hook in the rock ceiling. It was tuned like a Jamaican steel drum and helped ease them into meditation. They had propane, and Costco brand baby wipes, duct tape, Tibetan incense, a filtration device, and heavy black plastic bags full of junk. The only thing they didn't have was what they needed most: water.

Thick with poisonous snakes, mountain lions, and prickly cactus, the Chiricahua Mountains of Southeast Arizona are prone to landslides and are unforgiving to outsiders. Leaving the cave was an ordeal that left them exhausted and panting for breath. Since they'd arrived a month ago, the temperature on the mountainside had been unpredictable. One day it would be hot enough to melt the soles of their hiking boots, the next a freak snowstorm might coat the rocks, yucca, and scrub oak with a fine layer of ice. Scorching desert winds whisked away what was left of their moisture.

Despite the lashing from the cold, they thought a recent ice storm was a blessing in disguise. It might have saved them from dehydration. When he still had some strength, Thorson arranged a tarp to collect the runoff from the melt and funnel it into a water jug that was long since dry. They drank from the impromptu reservoir, and the dirty container of water sat on the cave floor, bristling with twigs.

It wasn't long until Ian began to feel sick. His guts cramped and he began to shiver with fever. He donned three sweaters and crept beneath a blanket to beat the fever back, but it wasn't enough. His face turned from ghost white to a deep shade of purple.

They had three things that might help stave off the sickness. First, of course, there was the power of prayer. They'd carved Tibetan words into a rock to sanctify the space and purify their spiritual path. Though meaningless in themselves, the syllables *om ah hung* in Tibetan invoked a powerful connection to their guru, which the holy texts said would restore their body, speech, and mind as well as balance the wheels of energy in their body, called *chakras*. Next to the carving was a course book devoted to Kali, the Hindu goddess of destruction. On its cover the bare-chested goddess clutched the severed head of an adversary and wore a skirt made of dismembered limbs. Kali is a fierce protector of her devotees, but she is known to take her payment in blood. Near the ritual accouterments was one more option: a sort of escape hatch if all else failed. Sheathed in orange plastic, the Satellite PersOnal Tracker, or SPOT, locator beacon was capable of sending out two prearranged distress calls. If Christie pressed the button marked HELP, their GPS coordinates would arc toward a geostationary satellite and into the in-boxes of their friends and family. A second button on the device, marked s.o.s., would summon the sheriff's department.

Christie stroked Ian's hair and it occurred to her that the illness could also be a lesson. Would he come back from the threshold of life and death with profound insight? Or would the journey kill him? Perhaps there was more to his illness than met the eye. It was entirely possible that he had been cursed by powerful black magic. She considered the tools arrayed in front of her. A protection mantra. The goddess Kali. An emergency beacon.

It was a test of faith informed by the fact that almost a decade earlier her teacher Michael Roach took her as a sexual consort and later as his wife. Roach was not the first white man to travel to India and come back claiming to be enlightened, but he looked the part better than any of his predecessors. Roach bestowed Christie with the Tibetan title of lama and ever since, hundreds of devotees bent at her feet. For them it meant she was a living goddess—a sort of messiah for a new breed of Buddhism that had only just gained a foothold in America.

Now that they were on the run, Lama Christie McNally had to decide whether she would try to heal Thorson with her godlike powers or leave the responsibility to an outsider who would never understand that the path to enlightenment is not always straightforward. Or safe.

As Lama Christie's finger hovered over the button on the emergency beacon, the stakes were higher than just life or death. Their very souls were on the line.

A Death on
Diamond Mountain

Part 1

Enlightened Minds

The First Bodhisattva

A Buddhist Parable

TWENTY-FIVE HUNDRED YEARS AGO *on the sun-drenched plains of India, a man who would eventually be known as the Buddha had a choice to make. He was thirty-five years old and had spent the last six years meeting with the wisest sages in the land, searching in vain for ultimate truth. Now he sat with his legs crossed, underneath a giant fig tree, with one hand resting in his lap. With the tip of his finger he made a slight impression in the dusty soil. After a lifetime of meditation, starvation, and pilgrimages to venerated spiritual masters, he had achieved something that no one else before him ever had.*

This was the moment of enlightenment.

A second before this, he had no answers to life's big questions. Why do good people die? Why is the world full of sickness and disease? Why do people suffer? But his realization put the universe in order.

Now he understood that every action that had ever taken place was intimately linked in a never-ending chain of causes and effects. Every living thing had countless lives. Good deeds in past lives brought good fortune in this life. Bad ones could bring disaster. The chain of action and reaction could take many lifetimes to play out; such was the law of karma. It determined everything in the past and the future.

Hindus already knew something of karma. But for them it was different: It was a tool used to justify a hierarchical caste system. Good actions in this life might mean a better rebirth. Ultimately, powerful people used their high position in life as a justification for their closeness to God. The people below them deserved their lot. What Buddha saw was more profound. A person could purify his karma and one day even escape from its clutches altogether. His movement rejected the caste system of the people who came before him and charted a new course.

This knowledge was power. And now the Buddha had options.

There was a way out of karma's straitjacket. Now that he had attained the ultimate knowledge of cause and effect he could leave the eternal cycle of birth and rebirth and enter Nirvana. If he did that, he would cease to exist; his body would simply melt away. In the ultimate truth, the world didn't really exist. For the people he left behind, it would seem as if he vanished from this world forever and entered a paradise where all of his actions were his own. He would be one with the universe. It was a pleasant thought and a just reward for a lifetime of struggle and concentration.

But there was another option. He could choose to live in the world and guide other souls to enlightenment. Staying would mean never stepping through the door to Nirvana until every other living being was enlightened. It could take all eternity.

No one knows how long it took him to make his decision. But Tibetans believe that he stayed. His realization made him a buddha—an enlightened being—but his choice also made him the first Bodhisattva: a word coined to describe the people committed to staying. Since then, there have been other Bodhisattvas and buddhas. Other people have attained similar realizations and instead stepped through Nirvana's threshold. All of them owe something to the Buddha's choice.

When the Buddha finished his meditation he uncrossed his legs and started walking to the place where he would give his first speech to a crowd of curious ascetics. The place he left became known as Bodh Gaya, which in the Hindi of today means "where Buddha went." He went on to lecture on the law of karma. And his lessons would found one of the world's most enduring religions.

Enlightening America

When the iron bird flies, and horses run on wheels, the Tibetan people will be scattered like ants across the world, and the Dharma will come to the land of the Red Man.
—A common misquote of Padmasambhava,
eighth century

MOST OF WHAT we know about the Buddha's life was first passed down as part of an oral tradition from teacher to student. It wasn't until four hundred years after his death, in the first century BC, that monks in Sri Lanka first wrote down the collected knowledge of the Buddha on palm leaves. Inked in the now almost forgotten language of Pali, the early canon is esoteric but is the best window we have into the life and times of the Buddha. Written down by monks with their own agenda for a unified Buddhism, the stories tell something about the Buddha's life, but they also tell us something about the storytellers. Later, as the texts went on to inform the political and cultural landscape of Asia, Buddhism carried the accumulated weight of history along with it. Each age had its own Buddhism, every ruler, scholar, emperor, and scribe adding their own perspective and twist on the ancient knowledge. The Buddhism of today is no different.

The very first reports of Tibet by Westerners mused that the monks' crimson robes were a relic from a lost sect of Catholicism. In 1507, Amerigo Vespucci, the man who discovered the coast of North America and for whom two continents are named, drew up a world map that plunked a Christian cross on the Tibetan Plateau. It was an early reference to the mythical Himalayan kingdom of Shangri-la, which Vespucci surmised was the home of Prester John, a Christian king purportedly descended from one of the three Magi who blessed Jesus. When Buddhism made it to America in the nineteenth century, it came to us through the lens of British and Russian colonialists who sent back curious texts, and images of deities floating on lotus petals. At the time, America was still reeling from the fallout of the cataclysmic Civil War. The unprecedented carnage shook many people's faith in God, and challenged their Protestant roots. New religious movements swept the land. Shakers and Mormons founded centers in the Northeast and West. Evangelicals predicted the coming of the apocalypse. And occult mystic societies rose in popularity. Buddhism and Hinduism added color to the mix of new religious ideas. Far from its point of origin, early American Buddhists filled in the gaps of their knowledge of the Eastern faith with their own Christian tenets. Like many faiths that cross over to new cultures, the result was something of a hodgepodge.

Now, several hundred years into the relationship, yoga mats, meditation cushions, and prayer beads have become the twenty-first-century hallmark of American spirituality. We play loosely with concepts and think of *Nirvana* as a synonym for *Heaven*, and Bodhisattvas as an analogue to angels. In doing so, we conflate two very different histories and religious traditions. The confusion leads to a dangerous conclusion: Buddhism teaches that it is possible to achieve Nirvana in one lifetime, and for some people with a Christian background who rush into Buddhism, it can seem like Heaven could be a place on earth. And no area of Asia is as romanticized as the once forbidden kingdom of Tibet.

Almost irrespective of the actual spiritual practices of the Himalayan Plateau, the West's faddish envy of all things Tibetan has spawned movies, spiritual studios, charity rock concerts, and best-selling books that range from dense philosophical texts to self-help guides and methods to Buddha-fy your business. It seems as if almost everyone has tried out a spiritual practice that originated in Asia, either through a yoga class, quiet meditation, or just repeating the syllable *om* to calm down. Today there are at least eighteen hundred Tibetan Buddhist centers around the United States and Europe. A further eighteen million people in North America practice some sort of yoga in gyms, private studios, and public spaces.

For many, the East is an antidote for Western anomie: a holistic counterpoint to our chaotic lives. We don stretchy pants, roll up yoga mats, and hit the meditation cushion on the same day that we argue about our cell phone bill with someone in an Indian call center. Still, we look to Asian wisdom in order to center ourselves, decompress, and block off time to ruminate on life's bigger questions. We trust that the teachings are authentic, and are the key to some hidden truth.

What we forget is that the techniques we practice today in superheated yoga studios and air-conditioned halls originated in foreign feudal times that would be unrecognizable to our modern eyes. They come from eras when princely states went to war over small points of honor, priests dictated social policy, and it was considered perfectly ordinary to send away an eight-year-old child to live out his life in a monastery. For people brought up in a mostly Christian environment it is deceptively easy to scoff at the preponderance of molestation scandals and liturgical hypocrisy in the Church, but far more difficult to see the same flaws in a tradition that they are less intimately familiar with. Many people are only vaguely aware of the long history of preposterous god men and false gurus whose philosophies have been laughed out of India, only to find success in America and Europe.

Even so, the East seems to offer something that is absent in the West: methods that join physical practice with spiritual searching. Yoga, meditation, chakra breathing, and chanting are powerful physical and mental exercises that can have a profound effect on health and well-being. On their own they are neither good nor bad, but like a drug that could save someone's life when administered by a doctor, they also have the potential for great harm. The traditions that are taught at home come from all across Asia and span multiple millennia, and yet we absorb them as if they were a unified whole, mixing together elements of Hinduism, Buddhism, Confucianism, and any other seemingly distant "Eastern" faith. The way we reassemble the spiritual practices of the East says a lot more about contemporary America than it does about their point of origin.

No concept out of Asia has as much power to capture our attention as "enlightenment." The English word derives from a time of great intellectual flourishing when Europeans challenged superstition and faith with rationality and scientific thought. It was made possible after the Greek and Roman scholars of the Renaissance rediscovered ancient texts in the archives of Byzantium. The Renaissance reinvented Europe, the Enlightenment refined it. Scholars in Europe translated the forgotten works and rediscovered knowledge that was thought lost. These textual explorers uncovered an abundance of literature as well as forgotten technologies like cement and optics. A technological and social revolution followed. The word for "enlightenment" in Sanskrit—*bodhi*—suggests an intrinsic knowledge of the world. Native to both Hinduism and Buddhism, its focus is on radically changing the self, not an aspiration to transform a whole continent. Yet the word we use in English brings with it the possibility of a renaissance.

In Tibet and India, *bodhi* is an ideal to strive toward but likely never achieve. It is a sort of perfection of the soul, mind, and body, where every action is precise and meaningful. For Tibetans, the focus is on the process. For whatever reason, Americans search for inner peace like they are competing in a sporting event. Here, enlightenment is the goal, and the reward is Heaven, or becoming a Bodhisattva.

For those unfamiliar with the term, in Tibetan Buddhism, *Bodhisattva* indicates an enlightened being who has understood the true meaning of existence so thoroughly that they have the ability to leave the ethereal plane and enter Nirvana. In doing so, the being acquires almost infinite powers over the material world. The Bodhisattva, however, chooses to stay in the world and help all sentient beings achieve the same realizations.*

It's no surprise that expectations Westerners have when under-

---

*People who are unfamiliar with the Hindu and Buddhist terminology can find usable—but to a scholar, no doubt, imperfect—definitions in a glossary at the end of this book.

taking meditation are often too grand. From a young age we in the West are steeped in tales of superheroes and Jedi who achieve great feats because of both their innate specialness and intensive study. We hear stories of levitating yogis, the power of chakras, tai chi and bad-ass Shaolin monks, and quietly think to ourselves that maybe anything is possible.

Some of these stories have at least some basis in fact. The Dalai Lama's own creation story was practically made for cinema. In 1933, the thirteenth Dalai Lama died in Lhasa and the reins of power fell to a regent, whose most important task was to comb the country for the recently deceased leader's reincarnation. After a prophetic dream, the search team found a young boy named Tenzin Gyatso in the remote Amdo province of Tibet. The monks presented the child with a tray of the previous Dalai Lama's possessions among a sea of red herrings. To the delight of the search party, the boy picked out his predecessor's glasses, yelling out, "It's mine. It's mine."

He was quickly brought to Lhasa, raised as a Buddhist monk, and anointed the spiritual ruler of a country. The story was vividly brought to life in the Academy Award–nominated *Kundun* and with Brad Pitt in *Seven Years in Tibet*, but also frequently in pulp fare.

For almost a hundred years it's been impossible to grow up without coming across near-constant reiterations in the mass media of Tibet's spiritual properties. Hollywood has capitalized on all things Tibetan since Frank Capra's 1937 adaptation of the novel *Lost Horizon*. In the film that came out of the book, a few adventurous World War I aviators crash near the mystical valley of Shangri-la. The inhabitants never age and protect the lost secrets of an ancient civilization. In other literature, merely showing up in Lhasa or an inaccessible monastery can inexplicably confer great powers. After Professor Moriarty killed off Sherlock Holmes in a climactic battle, Arthur Conan Doyle brought him back to life in his next book by explaining that Holmes had merely been traveling in Lhasa and Tibet for a few years. The trip enhanced his already formidable powers of deduction. In 1986, after the success of *Beverly Hills Cop*, Eddie Murphy played a vital role in protecting an enlightened child against demonic occult forces.

His travels in *The Golden Child* took him from Los Angeles to Kathmandu. When Christopher Nolan rebooted the Batman franchise in the first film, *Batman Begins*, he sends Bruce Wayne on a trip across a Tibetan ice field. The young superhero found a magical blue lotus on his way to a mountaintop monastery where monks trained him in martial arts.

George Lucas took great pains to see that Tibet would even influence our perception of interstellar space—the Ewoks in *Return of the Jedi* speak in high-speed Tibetan, and Yoda's philosophy and mannerisms are modeled on the Dalai Lama's. Luke Skywalker is perhaps the most archetypical hero who ever came out of Hollywood. Raised on a farm, the future Jedi had no idea that he was one of the sole conduits of the Force left in the universe. Through training with various robed recluses, he becomes the master of his own destiny and liberator of billions of souls. Two decades later, Keanu Reeves reinhabited the Chosen One spot in the blockbuster film *The Matrix*. Inspired in part by Tibetan Buddhist worldview, his character, Neo, learns that the universe he perceives is a computer-generated illusion; the actual world is a postapocalyptic nightmare. With a bit of concentration he learns that he can alter the physical laws of the environment around him, learn kung fu, and, yes, save the world. The role made Hollywood sense; six years earlier Reeves actually starred as the enlightened one in the film *Little Buddha*.

Eastern faiths seem to offer two diametrically opposed promises. The first is that it is possible to dissolve our overheated individualism through daily meditative practices, mindfulness, and contemplation. The second promise is that cultivating selflessness confers new abilities that, if anything, only add to an individual's mystique.

This is because, unlike many Western faiths, philosophy in the East is often interlinked with rigorous physical and mental practices that are carefully honed to change the self. While different traditions emphasize one aspect or practice over another, yoga, meditation, Qigong, martial arts, and any number of other activities have gained traction around the world not only because they are exotic, but because they work. Practitioners are not whittling away their time on aimless spiritual quests, they really do transform. Countless peer-reviewed studies show that regular meditation has a wide variety of positive effects. People whose brains are addled by attention deficit disorder find focus, the disaffected find empathy, and most people who practice yoga for even a short time report increased energy levels and an overall sense of well-being. Rigorous scientific studies that attribute improvements in cardiovascular health to meditation date back to the 1980s. Even the U.S. government has come on board when it teaches yoga and meditation in prisons to decrease inmate violence. Many insurance plans will dole out payments for acupuncturists and Reiki healers.

The trend is so pervasive that now it's common to find mindfulness in corporate boardrooms. Executives in Silicon Valley extol the virtues of focused meditation to help employees resolve disputes and become better managers. Mindful workers use their time better and report overall higher feelings of job satisfaction. The techniques help keep people in the moment and eliminate mental clutter. Physical practices build strength and balance—all good things.

The promise of enlightenment is a great leap forward from even these benefits. It's not about incremental improvements. Enlightenment happens in an instant, with a clear line demarcating the person before from the one after. As if transformed by the grace of God, suddenly the enlightenee realizes the true nature of reality, and the knowledge plants the person forever on a new plane of understanding. The mundane world is an illusion. After the first realization, various traditions teach that the enlightenment seeker progresses through a series of different eye-opening experiences until they reach the ultimate final state—call it Buddhahood, or Nirvana, Moksha, or some other type of transcendence. Whatever it is, enlightenment is also an experience. It is a sort of knowledge that is deeply personal and resists any sort of outside verification. That such a transformation is even possible requires a leap of faith. It resists scientific scrutiny and undercuts the very notion of a material world.

If we assume that it exists, then the actual state of enlightenment poses an interesting problem. What are people supposed to do with the rest of their time on earth once they've gained the ultimate knowledge of the nature of reality? Revered gurus who teach that status and power are meaningless in the ultimate reality nonetheless still have to muck about in the mundane world. They gather followers, build institutions, and dispense knowledge from lofty thrones. Is it hypocrisy when enlightenment simply reproduces familiar hierarchies? How does a Buddha remain in the world but not of it?

Still, we strive for a spiritual essence because we often feel that we are missing out on a vital part of ourselves. A person can live within the expected parameters of society, get married, raise a child or two, work forty hours a week plus overtime, and fully fund a retirement plan, only to discover at the end of their days that they failed to do anything meaningful with the years they had. There is no silver bullet for happiness, and living as a cog in a great machine of industrial global capitalism hasn't kept humanity's insomniacs from looking up at the stars and wondering what it all was for.

Humankind has probably always wondered about things greater than itself. "Who am I?" and "What is the meaning of life?" are perhaps the most fundamental questions we can ask. Enlightenment promises answers through mystical experiences and self-examination. Spiritual manuals penned and developed across dozens of different traditions offer specific practices that aim to form the body and mind into vessels for transformation. Training regimens take on many forms and can focus on extreme asceticism, or physical rigors that seem absurd. Or even dangerous.

It is as if the extremes are meant to reform a person from the ground up. Life, it turns out, is a preexisting condition. No matter how rigorous the technique, every person starts the spiritual searching from his or her own point in space and time. If every journey is different, what does that mean about the nature of transcendence?

Westerners, and perhaps Americans especially, have a conflicted relationship with danger. On one hand our heroes are entrepreneurs and adventurers who risk everything. We relish stories of the businessman who spends his last hundred dollars on a suit so he can pitch a great idea that secures a wealthy investor. We admire the mountaineer who puts it all on the line for a chance to summit an unclimbable peak.

But when risk takers fail in their pursuits, we cluck our tongues and nod knowingly about their hubris. Failure, and perhaps even death, may be the wrong yardstick to evaluate a person's journey.

Ian Thorson was well known only briefly in Buddhist circles, and more so for the unusual circumstances around his death than for any of the actions in his life. Looked at from one perspective, his plunge toward enlightenment is an obvious case of madness. Yet lurking in the shadows of the cave where he died are clues about the idiosyncratic reasons Americans have adapted Eastern mysticism to their own ends. More important, Thorson's own self-sacrifice begs the question, How much is too much to risk for a chance to pierce the veil of divinity itself?

2.

The Box

I am the clown.
I sit poised opposite my interviewer. We both wear suits.
He glances from the hair in my eyes to my resume.
I smile hopefully, I just brushed my teeth.
I ask, "do you have any openings for rock stars?"
— Ian Thorson, "The Clown"

KAY THORSON IS a spry and agile woman in her sixties, and her hair burns a fierce red. She still lives in a two-floor apartment on an outcast spit of land between Manhattan and Queens known as Roosevelt Island. The only pedestrian connections from here to the rest of the city are a single subway stop on the F train and a gondola that floats above the East River to Midtown. Like all islands, Roosevelt Island is a culture unto itself—in this case, one that has the odd air of a preplanned ski town that sprang up too quickly. Before the New York State Development Corporation took it over to create a bedroom community, it was a peripheral dumping ground for municipal projects. Known as Welfare Island until 1971, it has variously been the home of inmates, mental patients, a smallpox hospital, a single church, and a stately Gothic lighthouse. A lone diner called Trellis still serves some of the cheapest burgers and sweet potato fries in the city, and is the only restaurant of note. Islanders claim they have the best views in New York as just about everyone who lives here can angle for a vista of the river. This is where Ian grew up: in the city, but not of it.

Kay Thorson sits at her kitchen table flanked by three-foot lilies in glass vases. Behind her are shelves full of the sorts of abstract modernist sculpture that took hold of the art world in the 1980s. They are clay, marble, wood, and metal. Most are glazed white with pale colors filling in flattened spaces and highlighting ridged edges. They resist interpretation but give off a sense of uneasiness, like they want to change into something else. Of late, she has been going through a creative period and makes her way to a workshop fifty-five miles up the Hudson River. She spends what little money she has on art supplies, rare wood, and marble. If circumstances had been different, Ian might have been an artist too.

It's been almost a year since Ian died, and Kay has never stopped searching for answers. Though he moved out more than a decade earlier, papers and videotapes of his poke out conspicuously from the shelves, evidence of her search for clues that explain his drive toward spiritual matters.

Growing up, the Thorsons didn't talk much about religion. But if you press her, Kay will mumble something about being Episcopalian and change the subject. It's not quite the truth, of course. The Thorsons learned long ago that not everyone was comfortable around Jews. In 1938, Ruth Karplus was on vacation in Prague when the Nazis spread south and east on their murderous quest for territory and racial purity. Her cousins would die in Treblinka while Ruth came to New York aboard an American transport ship. Ruth, like her daughter, had flaming red hair and the sort of deep brown eyes that men find irresistible. Soon she was married to a prominent surgeon. She brought a love of skiing back with her from Austria and she went on to have a successful career as a designer of winter fashions—importing some of the first stretchable material for winter sports. The family cherished athletics, and Kay grew up not only skiing but also surfing off the coasts of Long Island and, later, California. So while their Jewish history remained locked in their past, they found connection to the world around them through nature.

"For us, water was important," says Kay as she grabs a heavy stack of photos and flashes through faded family vacations. In them Ian smiles broadly, with curly black hair and a stocky, muscular physique. In one of them he's a teenager standing next to his kid sister, Alexandra. They're both in wet suits, holding surfboards.

Both siblings attended the storied Trinity School, which was founded in 1709, making it the oldest educational institution of its kind in the city. John McEnroe, Humphrey Bogart, Oliver Stone, and Truman Capote all spent time at Trinity, as do endless legions of kids born to Wall Street plutocrats. Already blessed with wealth and social capital, students from here tend to go on to Ivy League colleges and after that land high-paying jobs that might allow them to send their own children to Trinity, which as of 2013 charged an annual tuition of $39,000.

Ian's teacher Bill Zavatsky, a poet, journalist, and eventual winner of a Guggenheim Fellowship, wanted to instill a writing instinct in his pupils, and graded his classes by the sheer volume of work they could produce—merely counting the pages.

It was a habit that stuck. From then onward, Ian always had a pen in his hand and filled countless volumes with his impressions of the world. He wrote on napkins and notebooks, in letters to his family, friends, and numerous girlfriends. His notes move between English, Spanish, French, and German, over all of which he had some command. Sometimes, when he edged into sensitive material, he suddenly switched languages as if to hamper his biographer. There are school papers and countless poems, videotapes, and 3.5-inch floppy disks. He painstakingly kept receipts and documented the minutiae of his life with the intent to one day write a book. Before he left Roosevelt Island for the last time, he gave the box of his writings and memorabilia to his mother and instructed her to throw it all away. His cumulative work meant nothing to him anymore, but it is telling that he didn't dump the archive himself. His handwriting deteriorates from neat youthful high school scrawls into what became almost incomprehensible scribbles in his later years. It is as if, for him, the goal of writing became less about communication and more about inner struggle.

The box sat on a shelf amid similar boxes of papers, bills, and art projects until after Ian climbed the gravel slope of an Arizona mountain and installed himself in a cave. Months later, Kay took it down from its perch and laid pieces of it out on her office desk. Wielding a pair of scissors, she began to cut up the documents she didn't like— excising names and e-mail addresses, painful memories and unwanted people. She spent hours, or maybe days, on the effort, but there always was more paper than she could ever get through. The resulting archive is incomplete. Some papers are comically mangled with L-shaped sections that remove the name of her former husband, or a particularly worrisome ex-girlfriend, whose names and details miraculously survive on the next document. Kay wiped her hard drive of ten years of e-mails from her son, and seemed particularly attentive to anything that mentioned drugs or sex. Especially in the early years of the archive, he wrote about both subjects copiously. It wasn't until months after I met her that Kay could see the box for what it was: a window into the transformation of Ian's psychology as he moved from an ambitious young man into someone increasingly consumed by spiritual wanderlust. Only then was I invited into her life to search through the records. Over the next year and a half, Kay would stay in near-constant contact.

Kay pushes the box across the table toward me and offers to go through its contents together. "You need me," she says. "No one else can read his writing." It was not exactly true. On his good days whole pages are effortless, but more often than not, interpreting the scrawls feels like reading a foreign language. In a way, going through Ian's materials is a way for Kay to understand her son's decisions and to order the chaos he left behind.

One document that stands out above all others to explain Ian's draw toward meditation is one of the earliest in the box, from when he was only eleven years old. A sort of diploma, it is a numbered certificate stating that Ian had completed four courses of Silva Mind Control, a meditation technique that grew out of the 1940s blending of psychological methods and hypnosis, and eventually blended into the New Age spirituality of the sixties, seventies, and eighties. It was later renamed the Silva Life System and the Silva Method, perhaps to

sound a little less ominous. Designed to give children and adults control over their bodies and minds, the Silva Method combines visualizations with hand gestures and mental exercises. Silva advises his
students to meditate every day. The routines train the mind to overcome its inherent weaknesses and to reach particular goals by sub-
verting the link between cause and effect. According to the Silva
worldview, problems in the world don't stem from external factors
but from individual perception.

The Silva Method teaches that if you can visualize your problems
in a different way, then you can defeat them. To lose weight, you
imagine a thinner version of yourself and project that image onto a
mental screen. To cure a headache, you set an intention to make it go
away and then count backward, all the while imagining the pain
leaving your body. For children scared of monsters under the bed, the
Silva Method posits that demons can be managed by visualizing the
giant monsters shrinking down until they fit into the palm of a child's
hand. Who's going to be scared of a pint-size boogeyman? Another
lesson, dubbed the three-finger method, teaches a student to press
the middle finger, thumb, and index finger together while setting an
intention and visualizing a specific goal.

The ritual gesture serves to create a bridge between the mind and
body. In India symbolic hand gestures like this are called mudras. At
later levels, the Silva Method proposes that eventually the accentu-
ated power of the mind can lead to astral travel and remote healing of
the sick. José Silva, who founded the method, says that these are the
very same techniques that allowed Jesus to walk on water and lay on
hands. Like that of many self-made holy men, Silva's background is a
testament to both his entrepreneurial spirit and his openness to the
unknown. Born in Laredo, Texas, in 1914 to Mexican immigrants, he
had no formal education, but worked away his youth as an apprentice
in an electrical repair shop. A tinkerer, he was fond of inventing new
devices. Eventually his business grew and he widened his interests in
experimentation to religion, psychology, and parapsychology, creating his method as he went along. In time he credited his own story of
pluck and success to his mind's own powerful capabilities. With ded-

ication he taught that anyone with the right mind-set can develop superpowers and succeed in business, love, and life.

The Silva course materials didn't make it through Ian's mother's document purge, but a corresponding coloring book that Ian's sister, Alexandra, filled out while taking the same course several years later survived. Her yellow, pink, and red Crayola drawings carefully fill in the pale cartoon characters with halos of energy around their heads in sudden bursts of waxy color.

It's hard to say how Ian responded to the particular lesson. What little he may have written has been lost, but the early contact could have been a beachhead for esoteric decision making. After Ian died, Kay threw Ian's coloring book away. "I just couldn't look at it any-more. It made me sick," she tells me. "There was only one thing in it that I liked. Silva had a great method to help you get to sleep. I still use it," she adds later, recounting how she focuses on her fingers and starts to feel drowsy.

By the time he was in high school Ian filled out his lanky frame with the athletic build that comes from paddling a longboard through waves on the unrelenting New York coast. Broad at the shoulder, he had piercing blue eyes and was fond of black-and-white saddle shoes that seemed more appropriate to an earlier era. His good looks made him capable of melting the hearts of the young women at Trinity. He was physically perfect except that his eyes were decidedly nearsighted, a condition that made him alternate be-tween glasses and contacts and which continued to deteriorate slowly through his life. Uninspired by the hard sciences, he drifted toward literature and contributed poems extolling Mother Nature to the school literary magazine.

He was close to his family, paying regular visits to his grand-mother, who lived in a rent-controlled flat on Park Avenue with her second husband, Hans. Both were his regular correspondents and of-fered their home as a place of refuge when he couldn't stand being around his mother and father. Gagi, as Kay's mother was known, lav-ished him with attention, listened to his poems, and encouraged him to travel and see as much of the world as best he could. His high school writings reveal a less idealized self, though perhaps a typical identity forged from New York's swirl of disparate influences. In one journal from that time he writes that, as "a city kid, some of my friends chose to sell drugs instead of Big Macs."

Ian's godfather, Jan Van Beusekom, owned a small cottage in Geneva that the family would sometimes visit during the summers. Jan had worked as a colonial administrator for the Dutch in Indonesia, overseeing factory conditions for indigenous workers. Of his godfather's time abroad, Ian wrote, "Western businessmen, stronger economically stood basically unopposed by the poorer locals." In Ian's mind, Jan was a roadblock in the way of rampant capitalism. Jan was a man of action and a father figure. From him Ian learned to speak French fluently, and Ian looked up to him as an early moral force who taught him "to accept his view that to look after others is to look after oneself." In time he took up Jan's sharp criticisms of American imperialism and diplomatic aggression. In a rare letter where Ian mused about his future career, he wrote that he would follow Jan's example and dedicate himself to social justice.

Jan stood in stark contrast to Ian's father, Tom. Ian and his father were strained in the way that many fathers and sons are. Letters between them were often stilted and heavy on instructions. Ian asked his dad to send one bureaucratic form or another, and in return he received advice on whatever career-oriented task seemed fitting at the moment. One thing that was never spoken about was how the cost of putting two kids through prep school and then college took its toll on the family finances. Though Tom was a lawyer, he seemed to gravitate toward get-rich-quick schemes to make ends meet. The box of papers includes several missives between Ian's father and a company called Laughlin Associates, which specializes in creating tax havens and corporate entities that are supposed to be nearly impossible to sue. It was protection that Tom thought he might need later if the schemes he had in mind didn't work out.

Having gone to one of the top prep schools in the country, it wasn't hard for Ian to gain admission to Stanford University, where he enrolled in accelerated programs in arts and literature. In his first year he pledged a fraternity called the Taxi, which was best known on campus for throwing an Arabian Nights theme party where attendees wore flowing silk pajamas as if they were in a medieval harem. His sophomore-year roommate, Saul Kato, drew dead last in the housing lottery with Ian, and the duo was relegated to the worst one-bedroom in the building. "Ian liked dark spaces, and he agreed to sleep in the walk-in closet," Kato says. The arrangement afforded a level of privacy for late-night rendezvous, and both men benefited.

Where much of Stanford was wearing buttoned-down shirts and getting ready for careers fit for the late-nineties Silicon Valley boom, Ian was bohemian. He rollerbladed across the campus's intersecting bike paths and from one adobe classroom to another. Like many people on campus, he experimented with drugs, preferring hallucinogens—mushrooms and LSD—as well as marijuana. Women gravitated to him, and he embarked on a mix of long- and short-term relationships. They may have liked the mystical side to his personality. "Ian was always sort of a seeker," says Kato, remembering that Thorson sought equal parts novelty and spirituality, even if at that point it wasn't in an organized manner.

During his freshman year Thorson met Ceren Osman (not her real name), a dark-eyed Turkish student who quickly captured his heart. After they had been together for a few months, she found him late one night hunched over a terminal in the computer lab all alone, the screen casting a white glow on his face. The font was so large that she could read what he was typing from across the room. "That's when he told me how bad his eyesight was," she recollected. He didn't want people to know he had so much trouble seeing, so he'd wait to work on his papers until everyone else was asleep. It was an embarrassment that he preferred to cover up. Feeling hemmed in by heavy frames, occasionally he'd go without them and try to walk around campus nearly blind. The result was sometimes comical, with him squinting to make out landmarks along the way and bumping into trash cans and other obstructions. Perhaps one of the reasons he enjoyed surfing so much was that the large shapes moved in predictable ways and hard obstacles were a rarity. "He was happiest when he was in nature, whether it was skiing or surfing, when he could make out the outlines of a wave or trail but not worry about the details," remembers Osman.

Ian's sensitive soul sometimes made her reflect on her own values. "There's a saying in Turkish, 'I love you so much I could kill you,' that to this day I don't really know what it means," she said when I reached her on the phone. "But when I said it to Ian, he was shocked and started crying." He asked her why she would want to kill him; the very thought of violence, particularly against someone he was in love with, curdled his soul. She hugged him for a long time afterward and decided never to use that expression again. "But even so, Ian was very sensitive to violence. Seeing anything like it, even in a movie, made him turn away and would make him upset." As is the way with freshman romances, eventually he and Osman drifted apart, but they made an effort to remain close. She promised him that if he were ever in Turkey, her family would love to have him stay with them on his travels.

"He was seeking something, and an element of that existed long before he took to any formal practice of meditation, yoga, and whatnot," recalls another fraternity brother, Mike Oristian, who would take trips in their friend Jamie's car out to the nearby Half Moon Bay, where the trio could surf before class. "He was a good surfer—not something you would expect from a guy who lived and went to high school in New York City." Together they chased fish tacos, cold beer, picture-perfect point breaks, and women. "The good energy and good times could wind any of us up, but I suppose we came to expect that Ian would always have a different take on things, march to the beat of his own drummer, as cliché as that sounds," he wrote to me in an e-mail.

In a creative writing class at Stanford, Ian enjoyed pushing the limits of propriety. It's not entirely clear whether he was experienced in hedonism or simply idealized it as an elixir of his own youthfulness. Sexuality was taboo, but also exciting. A block of prose titled "White Lines," published in a Stanford quarterly magazine, featured a prostitute snorting mounds of cocaine off a jagged mirror through a hundred Deutsche mark note. After getting sufficiently high, his protagonist, Rilario, "mounted her. She spread her legs. He came. She watched the lamp's reflection in the cleaned mirror shard flash on the ceiling. He rolled off of her. She sighed in relief." The story ends in a depressing morass of ill-spent innocence. It was a subject he continued to come back to.

In his senior year honors thesis in comparative literature, Ian approached the formidable professor and literary theorist Hans Ulrich Gumbrecht to be his adviser, even though he had never taken a class from the mentor. According to the department's policies, the thesis should aim to be a sort of "PhD dissertation en miniature," and at first Gumbrecht was hesitant to work with the untested student. Ian was charming, however, and when he knocked on the professor's door he explained that he wanted to explore the links between intoxication and spirituality in the nineteenth century.

Over the course of the year, Ian grew on Gumbrecht and demonstrated a keen ability to absorb complex ideas and synthesize them on paper. Ian took risks with his writing, crossing a line between the impersonal academic approach and provocative images that attempted to challenge the reader's preconceptions. He tackled Nietzsche, Freud, and Baudelaire. Through them he argued that the Europeans of the 1800s struggled to understand divine energy in two ways, first through theatrical acts where mesmerists and hypnotists amazed audiences with illusions and parlor tricks. When the audiences confronted inexplicable illusions, the performers on stage suggested that mysterious forces were at work.

However, as different acts were unmasked as frauds, philosophers and showmen looked inward and began to experiment with what became the first widespread use of opiates, alcohol, and hallucinogens. The chemicals opened up a door to new experiences that could make someone feel they were in the presence of God. He likened the nineteenth-century craze for intoxicants to the bacchanalia of the 1960s and 1970s hippie revolution. By the mid-1990s when he wrote his thesis, he believed that drugs had lost their luster among spiritual seekers.

At its heart, Ian's thesis argues that evidence for divinity fluctuates between two poles: external phenomena that can't easily be explained—at least by people in the audience—and internal experiences mediated by intoxicants. In both cases, spiritualists attempted to create the underlying conditions for mystical experiences. And yet, the paper strains against Ian's own impish desire to revel in his own taboo transgressions.

He writes, "Whether or not my impressions on intoxication in the 20th century are accurate, one cannot argue with the fact that, if I mentioned that I have just snorted three lines of cocaine before typing this paper, the reader would at the very least shake his head. The line between sobriety and intoxication in the 20th century is drawn in indelible ink."

The paper impressed Gumbrecht enough to let it pass with only a few reservations about its overall coherence. In his comments, the professor mused on what Ian's future might look like. "He is a very intelligent young man who, owing to the ease of his talents, might go extremely far. He may also perhaps never find his place 'in real life.' "

With those cautionary words Ian set off into a world that seemed to be tailor-made for a fresh-minted Stanford graduate. In the summer of 1995, venture capitalists roamed the campus, hoping to brush shoulders with the next billion-dollar idea makers. Professors pushed students to found their own companies. Sergey Brin and Larry Page had just entered a PhD program and their research on search algorithms would eventually spawn the company Google.

Ian's roommate, Saul Kato, who had been studying physics, felt the lure of easy money. He founded a computer graphics company just two years after graduating and, like other Stanford iconoclasts, lived and worked in a rented warehouse before upgrading to a swanky office. In a few years he rocketed upward through a career path, founding and then selling a series of start-up companies. Along the way, Kato hired friends from the Taxi to jump-start their careers. Other friends fell into the nebulous, but high-paid, world of consulting. They landed gigs at multibillion-dollar firms like Oracle and Accenture that were flush enough to hire students based on pedigree alone.

There was a moment before graduation when it looked like Ian might have a knack for business too. In his last year at college he ordered several hundred T-shirts in bulk and silk-screened designs onto them. They were meant to get the attention of any sophomore carrying a red plastic cup full of beer at any number of impromptu frat parties. In a few months he netted a little more than two thousand dollars. Where another of his peers might have built on the success and reinvested the profits, and eventually entered the tech and IT pipelines to financial liberation, Ian had different plans. He used the cash to buy a one-way plane ticket to Europe. It was seed capital for his world trip. From there he planned to just keep going east.

Before he left he spent a few weeks in Montauk with his family. The beach house was a two-story saltbox with few windows and a blocky floor plan. The Thorsons stored their collection of surfboards there, and it was just a short drive in the wood-paneled station wagon to the coast. Ian telegraphed his excitement for his graduation trip and pored over the complex nexus of visas, permission forms, and vaccines that he would need to cross one border after another. In a letter to his grandmother thanking her for a hefty cash graduation gift, he outlined a plan to cross Europe, Russia, Turkey, India, Indonesia, Japan, and the United States from California to New York. Kay remembers his excitement before his grand adventure. "It was all funded by earnings that he had saved, family contributions—not much, like a hundred dollars here—saving birthday gifts and such. Also he was determined to work, and did do work here and there, paying for this and that or contributing for room and board, either writing or translating on six-month stints where he could find it," she says, remembering the optimism in her son's eyes.

Like many a traveler before him, Ian planned to find, and maybe reinvent, himself in foreign lands. His family would hear from him only through letters and fax machines. The box contains dozens of letters from his world trip; most start out by expressing thanks for the continued financial contributions of the people at home. Occasionally they came with an urgent request for help negotiating one bureaucratic hurdle or another. The missives arrived postmarked with decaying stamps in unusual currencies—from Bulgaria and St. Petersburg, Ireland and Istanbul, Geneva and Morocco, Transylvania and from an ex-girlfriend's house in Sofia, Bulgaria.

While staying in the shadow of the Carpathian Mountains, he found a decrepit monastery where he hoped to find grace among the sincerely devout. While he was in town, he found a battered copy of a book by the explorer, Theosophist, and mystic Alexandra David-Néel, in the adventure travel section of an English-language store. In the mid-1990s, Chinese authorities routinely closed Tibet's borders to foreign travelers as they extended their violent crackdown on all things Tibetan. David-Néel's tales of sneaking into Tibet disguised as a pilgrim fascinated Ian. On her sojourn she met monks in remote Himalayan caves and reported back to her readers that she took magical initiations in secret smoke-filled ceremonies. She was transgressive in an era when women lacked opportunities and was an adventurer against all odds. Somehow she'd discovered something special in the highest points on earth.

Ian pored over the book in dark monastic chambers and he contrasted the Christian backdrop to what he was reading. The monks' austere routines struck him as mindless rituals whereas David-Néel's discoveries seemed primal and pure. The monks prayed, and then worked maintaining the monastery, ate, and then prayed some more. Where was the fun in that? The endless monotonous labor did nothing to quicken his soul, and he opted out of an evening mass. He didn't realize that his absence would irritate the monastics. The monks whispered that Ian's dismay might be a sign of a deeper spiritual problem. One of the brothers wondered openly if Thorson might be possessed by the devil. "They promised to wake me up at midnight for a special mass that would help with my demonic problems," he wrote in a letter to his family. Uncomfortable with the thought of being labeled with the taint of Lucifer, he scrambled together his backpack and left under cover of darkness down a snow-covered road.

This being Transylvania, local people believed that wolves, bears, and evil spirits prowled the road at night, and he spent much of the time looking over his shoulder. Eventually he happened across an-

other monastery, whose abbot had not heard about his spiritual afflic-
tion and agreed to let him stay. Despite the hospitality, this was the
end of his flirtation with Christianity. In his letter he said that the
experience taught him to "fear fanaticism and look upon religion
with renewed skepticism and increased caution."

He continued to head east, and the trip took a darker turn just a
few months later, when he boarded a train that took him to Tajiki-
stan. From Uzbekistan, in the provincial capital Samarkand—one of
the oldest continuously inhabited cities on earth—he planned to continue his journey overland. The former Russian states were still recovering from power struggles left over from the Cold War. Ethnic
conflict and wartime strife crackled through the air with the sound
of gunshots. At a routine checkpoint a cop shook him down for cash.
As he looked inward toward the rest of Asia he felt the chill of his
own mortality for the first time.

In the next town, he met a Tajik boy who spoke to him in pantomime. Ian wondered why he was alone and asked where his family
was. The child drew a finger across his throat and mimicked the jerk-
ing motion of a machine gun. Ian wrote to Jan that it was "the universal sign for being mowed down by automatic weapon's fire." It
was hard to conceive of such senseless violence, and the child's
trauma weighed heavily on Ian's psyche. "Whether I'm unharmed, I
cannot say. It has taken down my faith in human nature. I also never
thought that this boy from New York could ever feel so constantly in
danger."

The interactions made him rethink his plans to go overland
through the mountain passes of Afghanistan, where the Taliban were
seizing control of the state machinery. He turned back and booked a
flight out of Tashkent. Hours later he landed in New Delhi on an Uz-
bek airliner as the summer heat cooked the Gangetic Plain. From
there the Thar Desert extends for hundreds of miles to the south and
west of the Indian capital and cooks the earth beneath the former
princely state of Rajasthan and sucks what little water there is into
the atmosphere. The uplift from the heat-generated air currents
brews imposing walls of sand that sweep over the parched land and

coat the city in impenetrable dust. Delhites call the cyclical wind storms *loo* and lock their doors against them. Some people say that the *loo* brings evil tidings.

To escape the heat, Ian traveled north and east into the foothills of the Himalayas. David-Néel's writings made him curious about Tibetan teachings and he heard that the Dalai Lama was planning to preside over an important gathering in the small monastery town of Tabo. He bought a ticket on a dented tourist bus and wended his way along unstable mountain roads to get there.

The Tibetan Buddhist monastery in Tabo is covered in white plaster and had been in continuous operation for almost exactly a millennium. The Dalai Lama selected its birthday for the rare honor of hosting a *kalachakra* initiation for twenty thousand Tibetan Buddhists. His words would guide their meditations for years to come. At its most basic, the *kalachakra* is a teaching about the nature of time. Tibetan Buddhists believe that the movements of planets synchronize with the steady rise and fall of the human breath and the circadian movements in the body. The initiation empowers adherents to sense the planetary passing and to feel unity with the universe. The Dalai Lama taught that, through *kalachakra* practice, a person can speed up their own journey toward enlightenment and eventually Buddhahood. Ian sat packed in the throng of attendees and listened to His Holiness teach about the wheel of life. The speech was in Tibetan, but he could listen to live translations of the proceedings on an FM radio station.

The event struck a chord, and for the first time he mentioned an interest in Buddhism in a letter home to his godfather. Being in the presence of such a holy man put the wind back into Ian's travel-weary sails. When he wandered through the crowds of similarly driven spiritual seekers, a thirteen-year-old boy swathed in the maroon robes of a monk caught his eye. The child sat on a balcony, and villagers dressed in flowing striped skirts carried silk scarves up a steep staircase before prostrating themselves in front of him. They sought his blessing, and once the boy touched their heads, they turned away

without making eye contact. Ian approached the boy with the brash-
ness of a New Yorker. Why, he asked, did so many people bow before
him? The boy returned Ian's gaze with an unnatural dignity and replied, "I am Rinpoche."

The word *rinpoche* denotes an honored teacher among Tibetans
and, in this case, was an indication that the boy was a reincarnation of
a revered sage who, in his previous life, was the abbot of a monastery.

Ian delivered his response in what felt like slow motion. He asked
the child where he could find a teacher, and without hesitation the
rinpoche responded, "Tibet." It was unnerving to see a child speak
with such confidence. Ian's jaw slackened in awe. Perhaps this was his
path. In a letter back to his godfather, Ian wrote that he was still keeping his head about him despite the experience. "Don't worry," he
wrote, "American Individualism is a great obstacle to donning the
robes. I have met monks from many countries of Europe, and have
heard of only a few Americans. Tibetan Buddhism is quite refresh-
ing, it claims not to be a religion because belief is not a prerequisite.
It's a method of training the mind to achieve great bliss."

In one way or another he'd meditated since he was a child. Now,
at a child's insistence, he dropped whatever other travel plans he'd
had and started planning to go deeper into the Himalayas. At the
time the only way to get into the once-forbidden kingdom was to secure a tourist visa into China, and the Chinese embassy in India was
constantly vigilant for pro-Tibetan activists and very reluctant to is-
sue overland visas to foreigners. Since they took over Tibet in 1951,
the Chinese feared that even pictures of the deposed leader might
strengthen the resistance movement against their rule. The Chinese
government systematically eradicated religious leadership within Tibet and inserted their own monks in their stead who they could be
sure would be loyal to Beijing. Since then, the Chinese government
had gotten used to imprisoning activist foreigners for handing out
pictures of the Dalai Lama to Tibetans.

Even so, Thorson calculated that the best chance he had was to
travel overland, which meant first heading to Nepal and then cross-

ing a spindly bridge from there across the border. After a brief stop in Dharamsala, he boarded a dented green-and-white public bus to the border town of Sonali.

The journey took him along remote mountain passes and past the rusting carcasses of other, similar buses that had veered from the roadway and tumbled down into the ravines. Other buses had plowed deep wedges into the terraced farms and the drivers left behind their vehicles' crumpled husks.*

Ian's bus stopped briefly in Sonali. The dilapidated rest stop is little more than a sprawling checkpoint between Nepal and India. Drivers spend as little time here as possible as they offload their cargo and pack it into vehicles that are licensed to travel on the other country's roads. Bored customs officers sitting in telephone booth–size offices oversee the mess and stamp the passports of the few tourists who come through. From here Ian boarded a second bus for Kathmandu, a further ten hours away.

Exhausted from his journey, but eager to acquire an entrance stamp into Tibet, Ian probed the Tibetan area of town called Boudhanath. Here a domelike stupa topped with an enormous bronze spear marks the heart of Buddhist practice in Kathmandu. He took a room near Kopan Monastery, which was one of a few Tibetan Buddhist institutions set up to teach foreign tourists the rudiments of the

---

*By this time in his journey, Ian would have probably realized that traveling along Indian roadways is an exercise in faith in what is occasionally known in the Western press as the "Karmic Theory of Driving." Almost every new traveler to South Asia experiences terror as they face the chaos of Indian traffic patterns. Stretches of desolate pavement are poorly maintained and the right-of-way belongs to the heaviest vehicle. Buses send three-wheeled auto-rickshaws and white Ambassador cars skittering to the sides. They make room only for the larger blocky, and almost universally orange, Tata lorries that deliver the bulk of goods across the country. At night, drivers keep their high beams on, not so that they can illuminate the roadway, but to deter oncoming vehicles. Drivers are typically momentarily blind as they pass oncoming traffic. This is the norm. Seat belts are unnecessary. Far too many Hindus believe that accidents are not caused by the material conditions, maintenance, or the typical physics of careening steel and rubber. Accidents are karmic events.

The consequences are obvious to anyone who has spent time in a car in India: Death seems always to be only a split second away. The miracle of India's roads is that, more often than not, people get to where they are going unharmed. Cars set on collision courses veer to safety at the very last moment. At an abstract level, there is no obvious explanation for why one particular object collides with another. There are tens of thousands of opportunities to perish on every trip; what force creates a particular absurd collision? Believing that karma is the ultimate cause of accidents can be a strange comfort that reconciles and explains the chaos of everyday life.

faith. Here both Westerners and Tibetans in robes sit for daily meditation and "middle-way" practice.

For many years Kopan was the headquarters of the Foundation for
the Preservation of the Mahayana Tradition (FPMT), which is the largest network of Tibetan Buddhists outside of Tibet and India. Founded
by two eminent lamas—Thubten Yeshe and Zopa Rinpoche—their
growing body of Western students allowed them to spread the monastery's influence deep into the United States and Europe.

Eager to learn more about Tibetan philosophy, Ian enrolled in a
ten-day meditation course taught by one of the Western students. In
the Tibetan language the course was called *lamrim*, or "Steps on the
Path to Enlightenment"; variations on it have been taught since medieval times. According to some people, the basic *lamrim* teachings
on the impermanence of things, compassion, ritual practice, and the
stages of death are profound enough for karmically pure people to
instantly achieve Buddhahood.

The pages of Ian's pink workbooks overflow with realizations.
The teacher asked him to consider his five senses—sight, sound,
taste, touch, and smell. They are our only gateway to the external
world and are the barrier between our minds and external reality.
How do we know that they are not biased?

The Buddha began his explorations into ultimate reality from a
place similar to Descartes's musing, *Cogito ergo sum*, "I think, therefore I am." The Buddha went deeper than Descartes, though, when
he questioned the very nature of thinking. To understand what exists
outside of our five senses, the Buddha asks his students to first understand the mind. The key tool for that is meditation.

All Buddhists agree that the only constant in the world is change,
and that change inevitably leads to suffering. Young people get older,
love fades, healthy people get sick. Karma fuels all of that change, and
every person faces the inevitability of death.

The only way to end that suffering is to exit the cyclic routine of
death and rebirth. That is, to enter into Nirvana. What sets Tibetan
Buddhism apart from other Buddhist traditions—such as the Zen
Buddhism of Japan or the Theravada tradition in Sri Lanka—is that

while Tibetans aim to become enlightened, they don't want to enter Nirvana. Instead, Tibetan Buddhists aim to transform themselves into Bodhisattvas. Bodhisattvas don't exit the karmic cycle but choose to exist on the cusp between existence and nonexistence in order to help all other sentient beings. Once every mosquito, fox, human, demigod, god, demon, extraterrestrial being, slug, and seahorse attains the same state of perfect realization, then all creatures and Bodhisattvas will cross over into Nirvana together.

As Ian Thorson sat on the floor of the monastery in front of a golden statue of the thousand-armed god Avalokiteshvara, he wrestled with the nature of impermanence. One particularly powerful meditation focused on the inevitability of his own death. He didn't want to go through life without contemplating its ending, so he pressed his blue Bic pen deep into the notebook and declared, "_I will die_." The phrase took over the top of the page. Thinking about death should be a call to action. When he lost his life, what would he leave behind? What meaning could he create that was greater than himself? In the precious moments he had on earth now, what was the right way to use his time?

"I've never been able to have any continuous discipline except when I'm depressed, on the rebound from something, or trying to accomplish some goal. But then I go back to not doing anything. I can't even get myself to write every day," he worried. Faced with what he saw as his own lack of discipline, the daily regimen at Kopan was opening a door to a new approach to life.

Maybe daily meditations could allow him to come back to America with a sense of purpose. And yet, even so, he wrote that the necessity to accept "reincarnation and other related ideas keeps me from jumping in head first. I prefer literature to religion and Dostoevsky's _The Brothers Karamazov_ has been my most recent enlightenment."

The course did not completely sell him on the Tibetan religion. But he was still curious and turned his attention to finding a teacher in Tibet once again. He started by probing the Chinese embassy for the required permits and was elated when he received permission.

His plans were briefly set back when he contracted a bout of dysentery from tainted food. Gut-wrenching spasms took hold of his body and he got stuck in his bed for several days, making furtive retreats to the squat toilet. Instead of popping an antibiotic, he went to a Tibetan doctor, who offered him medicine—brown balls of herbs and sacred magic—meant to even out the elements of his body and restore his health. He was soon on his feet, and then on a bus toward the border crossing.

"I had asked questions of travelers, read books, copied maps. I was ready to go. Where? Not sure, but to Tibet and then see," he wrote to Jan.

He hefted his backpack again and donned a traveler's persona. He hopped on a series of increasingly small buses, but this time heading north from Kathmandu. The thick jungles in the valley gave way to terraced hills as the bus rolled across rushing rivers and cut past spiny iguana-back peaks through the green foothills. Finally he came to the shadow of Everest, where a spindly bridge separated Nepal from the once-forbidden kingdom. A lone Chinese soldier wearing green fatigues and carrying an imitation Kalashnikov glanced at Ian's passport and waved him across the border.

That night he slept in a bivouac sack with a drab olive tarp over him as he watched the stars. "And there lying down perhaps I cried, perhaps not, only thought this one sweet bedtime thought. 'I am in Tibet, you bet,'" he wrote.

The next four months of his trip are curiously unrecorded. The box of his notes contains a few hand-drawn maps and the scribbled names of monasteries, guesthouses, and travel times. It is as if the emptiness of the landscape erased his will to record his impressions. Much of his trip, though, seems to have been done on foot as he summited steeply graded hills and found remote caverns and villages. He met the occasional Spanish and Swiss-German traveler and drank thick butter tea. He sent no letters home, but made it at least to Lhasa.

When he crossed back over the Nepal border, he was ready to commit himself to a Buddhist path. He traveled back to India, where he planned to visit Bodh Gaya, the spot where the Buddha attained enlightenment beneath a shady fig tree twenty-five hundred years before. He wrote to his grandmother that it was a "necessary stop on the dharma trail."

From there he traveled to Sera Mey, a Tibetan monastery in the Indian state of Karnataka. He enrolled in another course in Buddhist philosophy, but the English translations were still poor, and he struggled with the same concepts he had encountered at Kopan. Seeing that Ian was an American, the abbot of the monastery, Jampa Choegyal,* advised him that if he wanted to continue his studies when he returned home, there was a monastery near New York City in a small New Jersey town called Howell where he might find instruction. Choegyal gave Ian two brass statues of the Buddha and a hundred boxes of incense to deliver there. It was called the Rashi Gempil Ling Temple, home to an American teacher who had earned a reputation for translating esoteric Buddhism into plain English: Geshe Michael Roach.

---

*In March 1996, the Dalai Lama announced that a popular god in the Tibetan pantheon named Dorje Shugden was an "evil spirit," and that anyone who continued to worship Shugden would have to renounce their ties to His Holiness. Most Tibetans followed his ruling without question, but some steadfast Shugden worshipers stewed and plotted revenge. The following year, loyal Shugden followers murdered one of the Dalai Lama's teachers by cutting his throat and stabbing him repeatedly in ritual points on his body, which were aimed at ensuring the monk a lower rebirth. The assassins also killed two of his unlucky attendants. In the years after, Shugden worshipers have been excommunicated wherever they are located. In 2008, Jampa Choegyal was expelled from his position at Sera Mey for the religious offense of continuing to worship Shugden. The Shugden affair remains one of the most fascinating modern conflicts in the Tibetan community and is sorely underrepresented in this book. Readers interested in understanding the medieval roots of the conflict should locate an article by Georges Dreyfus, published in the *Journal of the International Association of Buddhist Studies* in 1998 (vol. 21, no. 2), titled "The Shuk-den Affair."

3.

The Curious Prehistory of
Michael Roach

*The greatest business people have a deep inner capacity—they hunger,
as we all do, but perhaps more strongly—for a true spiritual life. They
have seen more of the world than most of us; they know what it can give
them, and what it cannot. They demand logic in spiritual things; they
demand that the method and the results be clear; as clear as the terms in
any business deal.*

—Michael Roach and Christie McNally,
The Diamond Cutter

BY THE 1950S, Phoenix, Arizona, was one of America's up-and-
coming economic engines. The city sits tucked away in the northern
reaches of the Sonoran Desert, where occasional sharp, rocky volcanic
hills pierce the sands and thrust upward hundreds of feet. Giant pillars of the majestic saguaro cactus poke up in clumps across the otherwise barren tracts. It was here that Michael Roach's father moved
the family from Los Angeles in 1958 to help build houses on the grid-
ded streets that today seem to extend endlessly across the desert.

From the outside, the Roaches appeared to have a firm grasp on
the American Dream. Roach's mother taught in the local elementary
school and she stressed education to her four sons. As native Califor-
nians, Michael and his brothers loved to be in the water, but getting
to the ocean meant trekking back to the West Coast with their long-
boards strapped to the roof of the car. They seemed like a typical

upwardly mobile middle-class family, but on closer inspection the nuclear family's idyllic appearance didn't last past the time Roach was in sixth grade. Both parents were hard drinkers and their tumultuous relationship ended at a time when divorce was still taboo. Perhaps seeking to order the chaos of family life, Michael turned inward and aimed at perfection in all things. By all accounts Michael was an exceptional child.

Pug faced and earnest, he was an altar boy at the local Episcopal church. Assuming the acolyte role to an authoritative priest introduced him to the transformative power of ritual, as did his entrance into the Boy Scouts' exclusive Order of the Arrow. Founded in 1910, the Boy Scouts are a staple in millions of American households, and stress self-reliance and solitary encounters in the wilderness. Their rituals draw heavily on Native American symbolism and are kept secret from outsiders. After Roach achieved the rank of Eagle Scout, the leaders of his troop dressed in feathers and war paint—what passed for Indian ceremonial garb—and called out his name in front of an assembled crowd. Other prospective order members were turned away.

It was an honor, but to grasp it he would have to traverse a ritual known as the Ordeal. Over the course of twenty-four hours, Roach took a vow of silence, ate only meager rations, and did symbolic labor around the camp. During the rite, boys who had already been through the ritual bound him with a rope and asked him to take an oath called the Obligation. Afterward he shot a bow and arrow, lit a sacred fire, and spent the night alone contemplating his role in the world. It was tame stuff, but other Scouts report that the solitude often comes along with a twinge of fear. At the other end of the ritual the boys feel they are part of something bigger than themselves. Some would say transformed. Being forbidden to ever speak of the Ordeal except with other people who had been through it set Roach apart from other Scouts. The privilege became a literal badge of honor on a sash he wore across his chest.

Based on his test scores and recommendations from teachers, he was one of only two students from Arizona to be awarded the Presidential Scholars Medallion that year. He traveled to Washington DC, to personally receive the bronze-and-gold prize from Richard Nixon at the White House. From there it was a simple step to land a scholarship to Princeton University, major in religion, and contemplate entering Episcopal Divinity School in Cambridge, Massachusetts, once he graduated.

During his sophomore year Roach learned that his mother was dying of breast cancer and the news radically shifted his priorities. The impending loss made him search for answers, so he took a sabbatical from his scholarly obligations and flew to India on a quest for meaning. It was an impulsive trip, he would later admit. The semester earlier, at Princeton, he took a course on medieval Buddhist poetry from Japan and he thought he would find hope in the birthplace of the religion. There was no plan to speak of; he just had to run away for a little bit.

What he may not have paid attention to in his religion class was that Buddhism had mostly died out in India a millennium before he arrived. Beginning with the White Huns in the sixth century, and culminating with persecution by Islamic rulers in the fourteenth, a series of invasions and conquests swept away once-flourishing Buddhist communities in North India. The only reason Buddhism thrived anywhere in the world was due to medieval and ancient saints who spread the religion to East Asia, where it took root.

Only a historical accident saved Roach's trip. In 1951 the Chinese Red Army had invaded Tibet and imprisoned or killed thousands of monks. Tanks laid waste to monasteries, and only a few resistance fighters stood up to the onslaught for more than a few years. The highest Tibetan intellectuals and scholars, including the Dalai Lama, escaped south and west to India and Nepal. The Indian government welcomed the Tibetan refugees, and when Roach came to India, they were still trying to establish themselves in their new country as permanent residents.

Tibetans represented the only notable population of Buddhists left in India. Tibetans practiced Mahayana Buddhism, which is a different form from the one that had once been popular in India in the medieval era. Tibetans stress tantric, or secret, teachings that other Buddhist traditions sometimes scoff at as magic. Nonetheless, Roach

was interested in studying Buddhism however he could, and he located a small village in the foothills of the Himalayas outside the colonial outpost of Dehradun, where Tibetan refugees had set up a
branch of Sakya Monastery in exile.

He spent several months there learning rudimentary Tibetan and
studying classical Indian music. When he returned to Princeton in
1973, he'd given up the idea of becoming a priest. Instead he spent his
time securing funding to return to India. When he'd raised the cash
he traveled to Dharamsala, a Himalayan hill station and the capital of
the Tibetan Government in Exile, where he began a more formal
course of study. Feeling that Buddhist teachings on impermanence
might be useful to his dying mother, he urged her to take the flight
and bus journey to the seat of the Dalai Lama and seek treatment
with a Tibetan doctor. She came, took the pills and potions prescribed
by the doctor, and together they studied Tibetan philosophy on death
and dying. She returned home and died in April 1975 in Michigan.

The loss struck the rest of the family like a wrecking ball. His
younger brother, John, disappeared for a while and spent the year
surfing monster swells on the Hawaiian shores. It turned out to be a
sort of farewell trip. At the end of it, he took his own life. In a rare
video where he talks about the subject, Roach tries to explain his
brother's mental state and how his mother's death wreaked havoc on
his family's cohesion, paraphrasing his brother: "I'm at my peak, I can
surf Hawaii," he said with his voice cracking, "so he shot himself."
Around this time, Roach mentions that he was "involved in an abortion," probably his college girlfriend's. The world was full of death.

It was a lot to take in at once, but under the tutelage of different
Tibetan masters, Michael Roach learned that the deaths in his family
were not cosmic mistakes caused by rogue DNA fragments or depression; rather, they were born of the eons of accumulated karma. A devout Buddhist might exit the cycle of death and rebirth if he gained a
perfect understanding of karma. An enlightened person would know
definitively which actions in this life will lead to good results in the
next, and a Bodhisattva could ease the suffering of the whole world
through knowledge alone. Enlightenment eliminated the gray area be-

tween right and wrong. If he were enlightened, Michael Roach could help his family and ease their suffering in this life and the next.

Westerners had gone to Tibet and India and returned wearing monks' robes long before Roach arrived, but by the 1970s few had spent a significant amount of time formally studying inside monasteries. Fewer still had taken monastic vows that would confirm them in the community. Roach could distinguish himself by being one of the first. At the time, the Dalai Lama had not yet gained global superstar status and was easier to meet in person. While he was in Dharamsala he asked the Dalai Lama himself for advice. The Tibetan pontiff advised Roach to study in America and meet an acclaimed teacher named Khen Rinpoche Geshe Lobsang Tarchin, who was also known as Khen Rinpoche for people who couldn't handle the mouthful of titles. The learned monk was taking over control of a tiny dharma center located in Howell, New Jersey, in an effort to spread Tibetan Buddhism to America. The Dalai Lama warned Roach that his prospective teacher would demand complete authority over Roach's life. In return, Roach might become one of the West's best-recognized Tibetan Buddhist teachers.

A few months later, Michael Roach clutched his bankbook with its few thousand dollars of savings and walked into Khen Rinpoche's studio at the Rashi Gempil Ling Temple in Howell. Roach bowed low before the man whom he wanted to be his teacher. He offered his devotion, life savings, and a plate of Tibetan dumplings called momos that he had spent the morning cooking. His body quivered with the fear of possible rejection. Roach offered up everything he had to the man he wanted to be his lama.*

The title of *lama* literally means "teacher" in Tibetan; in Sanskrit

---

*This statement is almost true. There was one thing that Roach couldn't offer to his future teacher. Diamonds are an indispensable symbol to Buddhists around the world, and particularly to Roach. In the Diamond Sutra the Buddha considered the nature of enlightenment and used the diamond as a metaphor. The Buddha compared the mind to a diamond, which is both the hardest substance in nature and perfectly clear. After Roach graduated from Princeton, a professor gave him a Thunderbird Roadster as a present. It was an ostentatious gift that reflected the way the young man inspired awe in the people around him. Rather than drive the car, though, Roach immediately pawned it at a shop in exchange for a small diamond. As he met Khen Rinpoche in his parlor that morning, he couldn't bring himself to part with this particular symbol of enlightenment.

the word is *guru*. A lama doesn't only teach at an intellectual level, he is a guide through life. According to Tibetans, choosing a lama is one of the most important decisions in life.

The rinpoche was in his late fifties, was wearing heavy horn-rimmed glasses, and had a prickly shaven head. He was muscular beneath his robes, a physique acquired by thousands of prostrations to his deities, most notably to the diamond-like goddess Vajrayogini. Khen Rinpoche took the savings book and frowned severely. In a gesture of absolute disgust, the learned old man threw it back into Roach's face. He scoffed that he didn't want money. He wanted a student.

The monastery was new and still barely scraping by financially. Khen Rinpoche could not offer Michael Roach a place to stay. Roach would have to find that himself. To earn his keep, Roach agreed to become Khen Rinpoche's personal attendant, doing his laundry, driving him around to lectures, brewing endless cups of tea, and keeping the financial accounts. The rinpoche instructed Roach to adopt a rigorous meditation routine, which was soon paying dividends.

A year later, in 1976, he had an experience while meditating on the emptiness that permanently altered his perception of reality. He recounts the story frequently in his lectures, the most common iteration being that, while he was preparing a pot of tea for his teacher, he fell into a deep meditation where time seemed to slip away. It was the most profound experience of his life, the moment that defined every one to come.

Almost forty years later, on a video now archived on YouTube, he described the experience this way:

> *While you are seeing that object you cannot be aware of any other object. Which means you cannot be aware of yourself. . . it is just ultimate reality and you are in it. There is no other perception possible. You can't even think to yourself that you did it. There are no thoughts . . . you can't even tell how much time has passed. That experience changed your inner being forever.*

He checked his watch when the sense of timelessness passed by, and it registered that twenty minutes had passed. Perhaps the tea had boiled over and splashed onto the stove. The vision wasn't over, however. Before he could move, he felt a beam of pure, clear light pouring out of his heart. It felt as solid as a telephone pole and he felt as if it touched every facet of the universe. Then, suddenly, images began to play across his mind. He saw the faces of millions of creatures.

You see the face of every living creature in the world, not just people: animals, insects, birds, worms, whales. All of them you can see in the same moment, but separately. And get this. On every world. At the same time. And you love all of them at the same time.

When that series of visions collapsed he saw himself standing above an entire planet as if he were whizzing by it on the wings of a satellite. Next to him he felt the presence of a perfect woman. Her consciousness was palpable to him and together they realized that they were responsible for the enlightenment of every living being below them. Though it happened more than half a lifetime ago, recounting his dreamlike vision still makes him tear up. As far as he was concerned, after that moment, he was only a few steps away from enlightenment.

As a skeptical outsider, it is difficult to know what to make of the vision. People with a scientific mind-set are averse to accepting unverifiable data. And yet whether it was a hallucination on the order of an LSD trip or a profound spiritual insight may not be relevant. For Roach the vision gave him purpose. He credited Khen Rinpoche's teachings on emptiness with opening the door to the insight. After all, it was *his* tea that Roach had been brewing. So when the elder abbot came to him with a new assignment in 1981, Roach was willing to do just about anything.

The thousands of monks and aristocrats who fled Tibet in front of the advance of China's Red Army arrived in India and Nepal with little except the robes on their backs and a few religious texts that they managed to smuggle with them. The great institutions that they had built up over a thousand years lay smoldering behind them, and for the first decades in exile their sole mission was to reestablish a semblance of their vanishing culture in a new homeland. To their great credit, they did so, through generous donations from the international community and religious fund-raising. Hundreds of monasteries popped up around India. Yet administering the new institutions remained a challenge. Monks, it turned out, are not the most money-minded people. Their financial records were scattered and disorganized, and some leaders borrowed money freely on faith without much of a plan to pay it back.

The Rashi Gempil Ling Temple was technically a satellite of the once-great, now-impoverished, Sera Mey Monastery. Khen Rinpoche hoped that tapping the faith of Americans would ensure a reliable revenue stream and help the parent organization stay afloat. He asked frequently for donations to put the monastery's accounts in order. The sums were small by institutional standards—thirty thousand dollars here, ten thousand there—but the money went far when he sent it back to India.

Michael Roach proved that he could keep accounts at the temple as he performed his service to his teacher. Khen Rinpoche thought that perhaps there was a way to combine Roach's love of diamonds with the business acumen that seemed to come so easily to Americans. He asked Roach to travel to New York and find a job in the diamond industry any way he could. What money he earned in the business he must send back to the monastery to help feed monks and build new debate grounds. Roach could think of it as a lesson in dharma.

He was initially hesitant to give up his training at the temple grounds, but his master insisted. So a few weeks later, Roach boarded a commuter train that took him from pastoral Howell, New Jersey, and spat him out in the churning cauldron of human activity in Penn Station in Manhattan. From here it was a short walk to the diamond district on 47th Street.

Hasidic Jews dominated the street and hustled from building to building in wide black hats, with tassels hanging from their waists. At the time, and to some extent still today, the district was the most important distribution point for diamonds in America. Jewels came here in secure parcels from Tel Aviv, Brussels, and faraway India. Before they arrived, most of the smaller stones had already been cut and polished for their maximum value, but specialized gem cutters in New York City still handled larger rocks that required advanced skills to process. With no idea about how to break into the diamond business, Roach knocked on the doors of various diamond shops at random, only to be politely turned away. For an outsider the diamond industry was hermetically sealed. Most Hasidics trusted only people in their own community to handle the precious stones, and Roach's spouting Buddhist theology seemed like too much of a risk. Looking for a break, he enrolled in a class at the Gemological Institute of America, where he met Ofer Azrielant, an Israeli documentary producer who wasn't having much luck getting his films screened.

To make ends meet, Azrielant founded a small costume jewelry business called Andin International with his brother while he was still living in Israel. The two didn't get along, and his brother had the idea that he could ship stones to Ofer in New York. A Manhattan branch would keep the brothers at a safe distance and maybe lead to some new business opportunities. Ofer dealt in fake jewels and didn't know much about diamonds. He took the course to learn how to grade more valuable stones. When Michael Roach saw the hapless former artist eyeing gems in their shared classroom, he sensed an opportunity and asked for a job.

"I thought he was joking," recalls Azrielant, speaking on the phone in a strong Israeli cadence. The notes of his voice drifted musically between Brooklyn and Tel Aviv. Roach didn't tell him that he was a Buddhist, just that he wanted to work with diamonds and would be happy to start at the bottom and work his way up.

Azrielant knew he was getting a deal when he hired a well-traveled Princeton graduate who was more motivated by symbolism than by dollars. Roach proved to be a hard worker, and rose swiftly up the ranks. Since Roach had been to India before, Azrielant put him in charge of acquiring raw materials for the business and sent him to Bombay, and from there to a small, crowded industrial center called Surat, in Gujarat. In this sleepy outpost the young monk negotiated million-dollar deals on behalf of the company.

At the time, the diamond market was segregated: One market was for high-end buyers, where rings and necklaces might cost in the thousands to tens of thousands of dollars, and the other was in what Azrielant calls the junk, pieces that were so cheap they held little more value than the costume jewelry he and his brother had shilled back home. Andin International's genius was that it envisioned a middle ground for diamond jewelry whose prices hung around two hundred dollars per item. Azrielant clustered ten or fifteen small diamonds into 14-karat gold settings that were cheaper than one big rock, and soon the jewelry was flying off department store shelves. The year Roach joined Andin, the company grossed $1 million in sales. The revenue doubled in 1982, and again in 1983, and increased until 1989, when Andin was reliably making $100 million a year. Some years the gross was as high as $250 million. And most of the diamonds sold by Andin passed through Roach's hands at one point or another.

Although Roach and Azrielant may not have been aware of it, the boom years of Andin coincided with the rise of a grisly trade in conflict gemstones in Africa. Warlords there used uncut gemstones to purchase and stockpile Cold War weapons that fueled violent campaigns against innocent people. Movies like *Blood Diamond* and countless magazine features show how weapons were used to enslave entire populations of defenseless citizens in order to mine more gems and buy more guns.

In Angola, Congo, Sierra Leone, South Africa, Rhodesia, and Liberia, diamond brokers indirectly provided the funds that slaughtered between 2.5 million and 5 million people. Arms dealers like Viktor Bout accepted payment in African diamonds and then laundered the profits through resellers in Israel, London, Brussels, and India. While many of those diamonds eventually found their way to diamond cutters in Brussels and Tel Aviv, many of the lower-grade stones were fenced through India. As the chief diamond procurer at Andin International, Michael Roach selected Surat in the Indian state of Gujarat as his primary source for diamonds. Surat, which supports thousands of low-end gem-cutting houses, was a key player in the trade in blood diamonds.* Roach started making frequent trips to the city and selected the choicest, and most affordable, stones by the thousands. As someone interested only in the symbolism of the stones, Roach most likely didn't think much about where they came from.

When he wasn't traveling abroad, Roach continued his studies in Howell with his teacher—essentially taking on a double shift and a three-hour commute to his day. To enshrine his commitment to the dharma, Roach took monk vows, shaved his head, and donned the maroon robes of the Geluk† sect. Beneath that, he wore a red sleeveless shirt with a high collar. A bright blue thread sewn along the hem indicated that he traced his spiritual lineage to Sera Mey Monastery, whose clergy had been exiled from Tibet and rebuilt the institution in India. The robes set him visibly apart from layfolk, and so too would the Tibetan name he took for ordination: Lobsang Chödzin.

The most difficult decision in becoming a Buddhist monk isn't an external one. To be ordained an initiate also requires accepting vows of moral conduct. The four most important vows passed down since the time of the Buddha are prohibitions on sex, stealing, killing another human, and lying. There are a further 248 vows that govern action in the world, many of which seem outdated in a modern context (such as the commitment to never put a begging bowl on a slope, or the proper way to fabricate a case for sewing needles). To break the main vows, though, is the equivalent of a mortal sin in Christianity and could doom a monk to an unfavorable rebirth. Roach took them all in the solemn ceremony as had countless thousands of monks before him.

Being a monk and a businessman at the same time required almost superhuman discipline. At Andin, Roach's salary rose quickly

---

*Surat's role in fencing blood diamonds has hardly decreased since the 1980s and 1990s. In the early 2000s, the international community instituted the Kimberly Process, a method of providing authenticating certificates for diamonds so that it would be theoretically possible to trace diamonds back to registered mines. Presence of the correct certificate would indicate the rock was bought from ethical sources. But the system broke down almost immediately. "Rough Cut," an article written by Jason Miklian in *Foreign Policy* in 2013, showed that Surat remains a key link in removing accountability from the diamond trade.

†The Geluks are the largest and best-known sect of Tibetan Buddhism. The Dalai Lama is a Gelukpa, though not technically the head of the order (that honor goes to the head abbot of Ganden Monastery).

to a peak of about $250,000, but Roach instructed Azrielant to pay him only $30,000 a year. The rest of the money was to be given as a donation to his monastery and funneled into numerous charitable projects. For the monks in Howell and India, the money was a godsend. When a corn crop failed at Sera Mey's agricultural estate, the clergy reached out to Khen Rinpoche for help. Michael Roach fixed the problem with a stroke of a pen. He also managed to further ingrain Sera Mey with the New York diamond industry.

While Andin was growing by leaps and bounds every year, there was a constant need for polished stones. Roach opened up a small workshop on the grounds of Sera Mey for monks to start their own diamond-cutting and -polishing business. This way Tibetans would be able to get a taste of the same magic that Roach had summoned. Roach's contacts sent rough uncut stones to Sera Mey, and the monks returned polished pieces. The business generated enough cash to keep the monastery running for a while. For reasons never explained, the venture failed after a few years. Nonetheless, everyone knew that Roach had boundless energy and was always experimenting with new things. Eventually other projects flourished.

Among his most remembered and revered projects among both scholars and the clergy was an effort to preserve Tibetan texts. Since the Cultural Revolution, tens of thousands of written commentaries by Tibetan scholars were at risk of being lost. The Chinese burned books with only slightly less efficiency than the Nazis. There were so few books left within the borders of Tibet that, at the time, the main repositories of printed Tibetan works resided beyond China's borders in the monastic libraries in Mongolia and St. Petersburg. There, at least 650,000 unbound books, each wrapped in a silk brocade, moldered away on archival shelves. Roach had heard about digital scanners while he was in college and figured that it might be possible to physically scan all the books in those libraries and preserve them for all time on CD-ROMs and hard drives. With a seed grant from Hewlett-Packard, he founded the Asian Classics Input Project (ACIP) and employed a small group of monks to man scanners and painstakingly enter every page of the books into a central database.

Academics embraced the project and it continues to be one of the most important modern archives for Buddhist scholarship. The archive gave Roach unique access to the most remote corners of Tibetan literature—obscure texts by forgotten sages mix freely together with more canonical works in the digital stream.

Roach's financial and social clout all but guaranteed his advance through the hierarchy in Howell. It also seemed to be a reaffirmation of his chosen status. Not only did he claim to have had meditative realizations that most Buddhists have only read about in ancient texts, he also seemed to be doing good in the world. Though he was one of many Western students who took up vows in Howell, there was no doubt about his value to the Tibetan cause.

He was successful enough that other students tended to look the other way at his propensity to editorialize ancient texts. The problem came to the surface in 1995 when one argument broke out that called some of Roach's commitments into question. In that year he self-published a book with his teacher, titled *Preparing for Tantra,* which was a translation of a classic text by the medieval saint Tsongkhapa. The book outlined a commitment to tantric vows, the necessity to accept a teacher, or lama, without question, and the idea that tantra is the quickest and best way to achieve enlightenment.

It wasn't the quality of Roach's translation that upset the other students—its message was fairly well accepted in Buddhist circles. It was the cover that brought Roach to the attention of his superiors. The main image of the cheap paperback features a photograph of an ornate Tibetan statue wearing a jeweled brocade and golden crown. At first glance it is standard gilded Tibetan iconography, except one thing is amiss: its face. Superimposed on what should have been the sculpted image of the goddess Vajrayogini is a photograph of a young woman. It seemed like a lot of effort to go through in the pre-Photoshop age, and a monk at Howell questioned the alteration—why would Roach alter a traditional depiction of the goddess? Roach quashed the objection, saying that it was his prerogative to make the cover look like whatever he wanted. But he couldn't stop the rumors that the face came from a picture of a woman he'd dated in high school. If it were true, it would be quite a statement against the Tibetan Buddhist orthodoxy. Monks take vows of celibacy, and a lover was not the same thing as a dharma teacher.

There's no record of what Khen Rinpoche thought of the cover—he died in 2004. But on the balance, it was merely an infraction compared to the great good that Roach was obviously giving back to the community.

The book helped serve as a sort of dissertation. Khen Rinpoche awarded Michael Roach the title of geshe, which is the equivalent of a PhD in Tibetan Buddhism. He was the first American ever to receive the rank, and only the second person in the Western world. On a technical level it would give him a similar educational standing as Khen Rinpoche and the Dalai Lama. Some inside the monastery scoffed that the degree was not thoroughly earned—that he had spent so much time raising money that he hadn't qualified himself with scholarship. Under normal circumstances the geshes have to complete almost twelve years fiercely debating Buddhist principles with other monks on monastery grounds—something that would have been impossible with his commute to and from New York, international travel, and multiple entrepreneurial ventures. The exception for Roach may have been unique. Even so, Geshe Michael Roach had earned the respect of the Tibetan orthodoxy, had been an indispensable funder of the reconstruction effort for ailing Tibetan monasteries, and was a great preserver of texts. Soon he would found the Asian Classics Institute (ACI), an umbrella organization to dispense Tibetan Buddhism to the masses. It would seem he could do no wrong.

4.

The Acolyte

Yoga can kill or maim—or save your life and make you feel like a god. That's quite a range. In comparison it makes most other sports and exercises seem like child's play.
                    —William J. Broad, *The Science of Yoga*

THE THREE JEWELS Outreach Center and Bookstore opened its doors at an auspicious moment for Buddhism in America. It was June 26, 1996, and three weeks earlier, more than one hundred thousand people gathered in San Francisco's Golden Gate Park to hear the Beastie Boys, Red Hot Chili Peppers, and Rage Against the Machine play the first Tibetan Freedom Concert. The performers strutted and belted out angry lyrics beneath a giant red, blue, and yellow Tibetan flag. The national symbol of the exiled country features two ferocious snow dragons with green manes pawing at a red-and-blue yin-yang. Many of the youths in the audience had never seen the symbol before. The mythical creatures telegraphed their defiance of oppression to the swelling sea of people in front of them.

Giant monitors punched home the importance of the cause with tight and unassailable facts. More than a million Tibetans had been killed since Chinese tanks rolled into Lhasa in 1951. Notorious prisons were bursting at the seams with what was left of the Tibetan clergy. The occupation had left countless monasteries reduced to rubble, and a whole way of life was on the verge of extinction. The eminent Tibetan scholar and Columbia University professor Robert

Thurman implored the audience to take action against the genocide. An elderly monk named Palden Gyatso recounted his experiences in the Chinese gulag. His torturers demanded that he renounce his allegiance to the Dalai Lama and shoved an electrified baton down his throat. The shock caused all of his teeth to fall out.

Still, Gyatso explained that his religious training had allowed him to maintain compassion for his captors and understand that they were suffering as well. During the saintlike display, some in the audience held Bic lighters in the air like impromptu prayer candles until their thumbs began to burn.

Later, as the music gained tempo, Billy Corgan of Smashing Pumpkins screamed, "Tell me I'm the chosen one," as rambunctious teens crashed into one another, threw punches, and fell to the ground in a mosh pit the size of a city block. MTV broadcast the concert live and the crowd churned beneath the glare of camera lights. Altogether, the images of brutalized monks along with good old-fashioned rock and roll galvanized a segment of America's youth to protest oppression half a world away.

Tibet was cool. People were drawn to the Tibetan cause for its obvious analogies to the Nazi Holocaust. They were also intrigued by its unusual religion. What made Gyatso so compassionate in the face of oppression? What made Tibetans so special?

Michael Roach was in the perfect position to answer those questions, but first he needed a place for people to congregate. Manhattan's East Village was the ideal location for a dharma center. Close to New York University and the historical home of the Beat poets, the Village thrives on its own eccentricity. It is a sort of cultural and spiritual incubator where a new religious movement can expect to find converts. In the 1960s the International Society for Krishna Consciousness (ISKON), known better as the Hare Krishnas, rented a storefront there. The small Hindu movement soon became ubiquitous. Shaven-headed devotees in white or pink robes chanted the name of their god in airports and city parks around the country. They passed out millions of copies of the Hindu ethical discourse the *Bhagavad Gita* and parlayed offers of free Indian food at their temples into pitches for inner peace. Over the course of fifty years, the Hare Krishnas grew to more than four hundred dharma centers, storefronts, buildings, and intentional communities scattered across the globe. Perhaps Three Jewels could do the same.

Roach's budding following didn't care that the storefront was ramshackle. In time the shop would sell spiritual books and offer yoga and meditation classes, but for now Roach used it to lecture on the Buddhist concept of emptiness. In the growing word soup of the organizations founded by Roach, the Three Jewels was the entryway to the Asian Classics Institute, under whose aegis Roach taught Buddhist dharma.* Roach's students began papering the city with flyers and reaching out to yoga teachers and meditation programs. Their selling point was that a Tibetan monk who had made a fortune in the diamond business would offer the keys to inner peace, love, and financial success. The lectures were free. Roach had already tacked on the title *geshe* to his name, and the distinction helped draw interest from every quarter of Manhattan. It wasn't difficult to fill the shop.

On the opening night, the room was crowded and damp with the curious bodies of teens and twentysomethings. In addition to the new crowd, there were many familiar faces in the audience who had listened to Roach's lectures in New Jersey and in public parks around Manhattan. The older students instructed newcomers to pay respect to the holy space by removing their shoes before entering. The small shoe rack by the door proved to be inadequate for its job. A mound of sandals, socks, and sneakers overflowed onto the floor. A framed picture of the Dalai Lama smiled benevolently out at the room from above the pile. He seemed to look sideways at the stage Michael Roach would soon occupy. The crowd hummed with electricity as the anticipation grew. They shifted on maroon meditation cushions; some clutched the stems of flowers in their hands. The wait felt interminable.

---

*Not to be confused with the Asian Classics Input Project (ACIP), which Roach founded to digitally preserve Tibetan texts; the Diamond Cutter Institute (DCI), which exists to give business executives Buddhist tips on accumulating wealth; the Star in the East (SITE), which attempts to unify Christian and Buddhist philosophies; or even Diamond Mountain University (DMU), which eventually became the centerpiece for Roach's activities. Roach's multiple organizations lack a central unifying body except, perhaps, his own charisma.

The murmur hushed when an attendant swished open the front door to the bookshop and cleared the way as Michael Roach entered from the street. Clad in maroon robes, he bowed from his hunched shoulders and kept his palms pressed together. His hair was short and boy-cropped with a part down the side. It wasn't the shorn scalp of a monk. It projected a more get-down-to-business-in-the-boardroom air. The audience hastily cleared an aisle to the stage. With every step, someone new pressed a red, white, or yellow carnation into his hand. He nodded and smiled at them. Occasionally he leaned in close and whispered a secret or a pleasantry into an ear. A few were overcome and elated at the proximity to a person they considered holy. They beamed exaggerated grins as he passed and moved on to the next devotee. When his hands were full of green stems, he passed the flowers to the two women in his wake. In another context they might have been sisters, both with long brown hair falling past their shoulders and pleasant smiles. And like many sisters, one got the lion's share of the attention. More eyes gravitated to Christie McNally than to Mercedes Bahleda. The women were attentive to the geshe's every move. As he took the stage, they arranged the flowers on an altar off to the side. The blossoms framed the images of the Buddha as well as the pictures of Roach's own teachers in India and New Jersey.

Making a show of sitting down, Roach fussed with his robes and arranged them on his lap. It was a routine he'd seen monks do for years, a sort of absentminded and unconcerned romp of fabric. As he flattened the folds of the crimson material, students who had been there before clasped their hands over their heads and bent forward and then onto their knees and prostrated themselves almost flat on the ground. It was a sign of respect as old as Buddhism itself. For those who found wisdom in his teachings, it was a symbol of their devotion.

Before anyone said a word, Roach signaled the beginning of his talk by folding his hands into a mudra—a sort of ritualized knot of fingers that to the uninitiated might resemble a gang sign in another context. Though there are dozens, if not hundreds, of possible mudras, this particular one was meant to represent an offering to divine wisdom.

The effect is supposed to imitate the Buddhist map of the universe in the same way that citizens from Michigan and Wisconsin use their palms to explain their state's geography. Roach, and the students who could figure it out, intertwined their digits in a crisscross pattern to signify the four continents of Tibet's medieval conception of the world. In the middle, their ring fingers stood straight up to symbolize Mount Meru. In the Tibetan cosmology, Mount Meru occupies the same position as Mount Olympus did to the ancient Greeks, as home of the divine pantheon. A few people began to chant in Tibetan. Students who were new to the group were easy to spot as they fumbled clumsily with the complex gestures and chants. The ritual played out that way every time the group gathered. Only when it was complete did Michael Roach clear his throat and begin to talk.

His voice had an odd way of fluctuating as he paused pregnantly, or squirreled to a higher octave as he punctuated his points. The aim of the lecture wasn't always easy to discern through philosophical asides, references to pop culture, and inside jokes about Buddhist masters. Since this was one of the first meetings at the new dharma center, he wanted to be sure the audience grasped the most fundamental concept of his faith. For this lesson he needed a prop. He reached inside the yellow vest he wore under his robe and pulled out a pen, letting it quiver between his index and middle fingers in front of the audience.

"This is all you need to understand emptiness," he said as he began the routine he'd practiced at the monastery in Howell and perfected in lectures around the city before the official opening of the Three Jewels. "There is no pen here," he began provocatively. "There is a stick. It is purple, and it has a rounded shape. But what you're looking at right now is not *a pen*. You are seeing *Pen*."

Half the audience smiled knowingly. The faces of the other half were blank. Roach clarified with a question.

"To you this is a pen, but what would it be to a dog?" he asked with a cocked eyebrow. "A dog can't write. It doesn't care about pens. For the dog it is a chew toy." As the thing in his hand transformed from a pen to a chew toy in their minds, more people smiled. "For you it is a pen, for the dog it is a toy, but how can it be both? The idea for Pen does not come from its own side. That knowledge must come from somewhere else. It's coming from you."

This concept of emptiness lies at the foundation of much of Tibetan Buddhism. Roach explained that the pen was *empty* of any intrinsic value or meaning. The knowledge of what a pen is begins in the primordial soup of the mind.

What followed was a philosophical discourse on the nature of reality. Plato, Aristotle, and countless scribes, scholars, and mystics through the ages have wrestled with the problem. Tibetans have chewed on it for millennia. Descartes reasoned that the common denominator of human experience was thought and that since thought was irrefutably real, then the mind that thought the thought had to be real too. Therefore the world must also be real.

For his part, Plato believed that all objects are mere shadows of an elementary ideal type. All trees were imperfect copies of an ideal tree, and we recognize all trees through their "tree-ness." The same holds true for dogs and "dog-ness" or even cups and their "cup-ness." For Plato these ideal forms were not imaginary objects, but real ones that floated around in an ethereal empirical realm that existed beyond the direct perception of humans.

Roach built his version of Tibetan Buddhism on Plato's conception of reality and then took it one step further. Perhaps there *is* no real world at all. There is no way to know if what we sense actually exists. Sensing, in itself, is problematic. Every feeling, taste, touch, and emotion has to first break through the barrier of our skin, blood, and neurons. The flesh-sack filter touches everything, and on a profound level, who is to say that the mind itself isn't simply inventing the idea of a body in the first place?

Everything that we think we know—from the smallest atom and subquark to the planets and solar systems that make up the heavens, and even the brain matter that processes information—might just be a hologram of some even more profound reality. After all, what do we really know about the world outside of our own minds?

Once that thought sank in, Roach offered up another idea. Perhaps, if you change your own mind, the world will change along with it.

Roach gesticulated with the purple tube of ink and plastic and thrust it into the air. "When you can understand the difference between *a pen* and *Pen* you can transform yourself completely. You could be an angel." It is as simple as that.

When Ian Thorson flew back from Asia, it wasn't on the wings of an angel, but as a ticketed passenger on a 747 jetliner. The last stop on his trip had been Indonesia, where he met an old surfing buddy from Stanford. By that time, after almost two years on the road, Ian was more expressive about his budding spirituality and inquisitive about finding new ways to view the world. On one expedition, he searched out a sacred cow and hoped it might be able to help cure his poor eyesight. He knelt in front of it, prayed, and allowed it to lick his eyes. It didn't work, and Thorson later admitted to his friend Mike Oristian that "it was a long way to go to have the feeling of sandpaper on his eyes."

His world tour ended with a flight home to New York, the same city he had started in. But he was determined to find something that would give him more direction than a sacred cow, to find a Buddhist teacher who could further the training he began in India and Tibet.

At the bottom of his rucksack, he carried the gifts he'd received at Sera Mey along with instructions to deliver them to the temple in Howell. It turned out that he didn't need to go all that way; his spiritual progress was only a subway ride away. Michael Roach had just established the Three Jewels Outreach Center, and the buzz around New York was that this man really understood emptiness. After more than a year furiously scribbling out notes and letters to family and friends, Ian's first interactions with Michael Roach are curiously absent from the records he left behind. It was as if he was so absorbed in the new thoughts that he didn't have the energy to process the ideas. But what is apparent is that when he finally heard Michael Roach lecture on the law of karma, things began to click in a way that they never had during his meditations in India and Nepal.

Ian moved back into the same room he had occupied in high school, sleeping on his short single bed. The retreat to his parents' house underscored the difference between his own progress in a career and the success of his classmates at Trinity and Stanford. He was well traveled but hadn't made much of a mark for himself. Fresh off his world trip, the people at Three Jewels understood him in a way that his parents on Roosevelt Island could not.

It was still the height of the tech boom, and Ian's Stanford frat mates were making millions starting companies and selling them to venture capitalists. Ian consoled himself that none of them were transforming themselves into angels. Michael Roach promised the keys to Heaven.

Most Buddhists agree that meditation is the most profound act that a human can undertake to understand themselves and the world around them. Though there are different arguments about the nature of reality, the irrefutable common denominator of human existence is that we are all bound by the constraints of our minds. At its most basic, meditation is a tool for examining the mind.

For someone who has never tried to meditate, explaining the experience can be difficult. The simplest meditation is to focus on one's own breathing. Try it if you like. Feel the air move in and out of your lungs and try to stop the internal chatter of your mind. Try not to have a thought or let your mind wander from the sensation of breathing. Most people are shocked at how incredibly difficult it is to think about nothing. It can feel almost impossible to shut down that internal monologue. When this happens, teachers suggest that the meditator should try to take an outsider's view of their own thoughts. They should keenly observe their own mind as it spins out one thought after another. Sometimes, instead of focusing on breathing, you can focus on a single syllable, such as *om*. Every time a new thought comes up, focus on the sound and watch as thoughts arise and fall away.

In such isolation, it is hard to escape the sheer strangeness of one's own mind. Light patterns reflect oddly off walls, you might feel your heart beat in your chest in an unfamiliar way, or sometimes visions of swirling colors will spontaneously play across your field of view. With training and dedication, meditation helps disconnect the world that we take for granted and the world we project unconsciously. It can be tremendously relaxing and lead to profound insights. In the hubbub of New York, meditation might calm the urban chaos, or at least keep some of it at bay. It's surprisingly difficult work, but Ian excelled at it.

Within days of his arrival, his mother knew that Ian was changing. He'd wake up at the crack of dawn and abandon the idea of breakfast except for a small cup of tea. Then he sat alone on the floor of his room with his legs folded over each other in a lotus position, his curly black hair cascading over his back and shoulders.

He'd sit for six-hour stretches and then leave for an afternoon or evening meeting at the Three Jewels. His mind was changing, and he knew that he was better for it. Kay thought he should eat more and maybe, after two years on the road, start looking for a job.

Just a few months after his first class, he wrote a letter to his godfather, Jan, about how Roach was giving him tools to fundamentally reorganize his worldview.

> *I have fallen in love with these classes, which sometimes mirror my mind and improve it. I am slightly convinced that no matter where I am in the world I will not be happy unless my head is screwed on well. In class they have screwdrivers and hacksaws and bolts and butterfly nuts and bandsaws and hands on practice for head-screwing-on nicely. Actually it's logic, meditation and philosophy.*

Michael Roach lectured incessantly. At the inaugural lecture at the bookstore, he was just getting started. Though he said the world was empty of any intrinsic meaning, meditators can't help but notice that their minds keep churning new thoughts, which arise and dissipate on their own. Where did those thoughts come from? To explain their origin, Roach offered the Buddha's example drawn out of the natural world. Where plants grow from tiny seeds, so do human actions. In his book *The Karma of Love*, Roach describes seeds this way:

There are seeds in our mind, karmic seeds. They lay deep in our subconscious, deep down in the mind, and when the time is ready they crack open like a seed for a tree. I hold a black stick up in front of your face and in that microsecond a karmic seed splits open and out pops a luminous image of a pen—so fast that you've never in your life noticed that it was happening—and then you see a pen.

Every perception depends on a karmic seed, and every action that a person takes plants new seeds that crack open at a later date. Planting and cracking open karmic seeds is the fuel that keeps the cosmos running in an eternal hamster wheel. One action begets another.

According to Roach, the physical world does not exist in the way most people think of it. What we experience in life is the cumulative result of all our previous actions combined with whatever intention we have. For Roach, karma is a force in the universe in the same way that magnetism is. Unlike the forces of nature, however, karma resides in the consciousness of living things.

Good deeds in the present beget good results in the future. Bad deeds equal bad results. So if your lover dumps you and breaks your heart, the karmic cause could have been that you hurt an animal in your last life. The karmic seeds of hurting the animal lay dormant until, for whatever reason, the ground was right to mature. Meanwhile, if you helped someone in a past life get a job, that seed might ripen into a good career in this one. The goal of Buddhism, though, is to eliminate karma entirely: to clean the slate of all karmic seeds so that no action is determined by the past. Enlightenment means freedom from karma. No seeds means liberation from the straitjacket of prior actions. A person can become pure essence, where the mind would be as pure and hard as a flawless diamond.

The Buddha taught that there are two routes to enlightenment: One is slow and safe, the other fast and dangerous. The first path is called sutra, which is a system of open teachings that anyone is allowed to learn. Sutras teach a person to manage their karmic seeds by living a conscious and compassionate life. It focuses on ethics and addresses the way a society should function together. Sutra followers

slowly remove themselves from the world and try to leave as little
mark as possible on the things around them. By being a good person
and taking slow, meaningful conscious actions, a person—or, rather,
their mind—should be able to eliminate all their karma and become
a Buddha. The only catch is that the process is painfully slow. The
Buddha taught that it would take thousands, or even millions, of lifetimes to clear out past karma simply through conscious action alone.

The second path is called tantra, meaning "secret," and is considered so treacherous that only students who have mastered the sutra
teachings are allowed to learn it. In tantra, a person connects directly
with divine energy to burn up karmic seeds. Where followers of the
sutras try to tame their passions, tantrics stoke their flames and try to
learn how even extreme emotional states are also by nature empty.
Tibetans teach that the energy generated from tantric practice is so
powerful that a devout adherent should be able to reach enlightenment in a single lifetime.

Where sutra develops a person to be well adjusted in society at
large, tantra is a more individual path. Tantrics look inward and
change their own minds instead of acting in the world itself.

When Ian arrived at the bookshop, Michael Roach was teaching
the sutras. However, the promise of tantra was on the horizon. The
full course of sutra teachings would take seven years, Roach told
them, but once they had mastered his teachings and given themselves
over to him as their guru, Heaven would be within reach.

The walls of the bookstore were crowded with the colorful statues and paintings of Tibetan deities. Some of the gods clutched the
severed heads of their enemies while wreathed in orange flames, others cast benevolent smiles cryptically downward. One painting de-
picted a woman with full breasts wearing a garland of human skulls.
The goddess balanced a spear delicately on her shoulders and lifted a
conch shell full of ambrosia to her lips. Her three eyes grimaced men-
acingly upward and the shaven lips of her vagina were open and in-
viting. The goddess was Vajrayogini, the deity that Michael Roach
credits for bringing him to the cusp of enlightenment.

The paintings, known as *tangkas*, are aids for meditation and are considered by Tibetans to be emanations of the gods themselves. They look menacing, or benevolent, and to the uninitiated they are little more than impenetrable works of art. To understand the mudras and the symbolic language hidden inside each painting, students must take private classes with the guru. Students must promise not to reveal the secret meanings of the art to people who have not gone through tantric initiation, or risk thousands of years of torment in hellish rebirths.

Ian was curious about how the symbolic landscape and obscure movements of a deity could open up a secret world of meaning, and Roach seemed to be what he was looking for. The American monk was charismatic and could explain the esoteric ideas while at the same time quipping a joke. In his search to understand more, Ian became a fixture at the center and wanted to dedicate as much time to helping the group succeed as possible. It also seemed to help that the center was a magnet for attractive women.

Inside the Three Jewels, physical contact was a given. Vibrant and young women gave him hugs when he walked through the door, and Roach gave lectures on the nature of sexuality that piqued Ian's interest. After he'd been in classes for about a month, he began to type out a letter on his laptop while he sat on a grimy train platform. It was addressed to his friend LaShaun Williams in Baltimore. They had met at Stanford and now LaShaun was studying to be a psychologist. They were both interested in the esoteric side of the human mind.

There are these two girls that are constantly around me, one who works on my patience the other on my desire. It's really kind of incredible but I feel like I have not been alone in so, so long. It's a feeling that I am not used to having. Anyhow, we just had a really long class on the value of celibacy that me and my involved-with-lady attended. It's pretty heavy and I buy all of it, basically if you were properly trained to channel all of the energy used for sex into some intense self-transformative exercises, you would not even consider having sex. It would be so much less fun than what you were doing. But what about in the meantime when you were not yet trained, who knows, right?

Within a few weeks Ian was spending much of his time with Roach's two closest attendants: Christie McNally and Mercedes Bahleda. The duo hung on Roach's every word and exuded the effortless love and kindness that was de rigueur to recruiting new members. Both had troubled pasts.

Bahleda grew up in a bucolic village on the outskirts of Buffalo, New York, called Hamburg. She was the daughter of a Catholic school art teacher who was bringing up two daughters alone. In 1977, when Mercedes was still just a girl, a sixteen-year-old recluse broke into the house with a crowbar and bludgeoned her mother to death with it. In the morning, Mercedes and her sister came downstairs and found their mother's bloodied corpse. The crime was without apparent motive.

Bahleda's father, James, was the initial suspect, and the police investigation ripped the already fragile family apart and left him under a cloud of suspicion. It wasn't until seventeen years later that the cops arrested another man for arson and he accidentally confessed to the murder.

Bahleda was never the same. Both she and her sister endured years of psychological counseling, but nothing seemed to explain how such evil could exist in the world, or why her mother was so cruelly ripped away from her. She sought explanations, and there was something soothing in Roach's teachings that created order. Something that her mother had done in the past—probably a past life—had predicted her murder. Mercedes's karma was to find the body and grow up in a broken home.

Now that she was at the Three Jewels, Mercedes seemed to have come to terms with the death. Roach's explanations helped soothe the pain, and gave her the strength to take control of the damage that had been a scourge of her childhood. Meditation helped her scour away the bad karmic seeds and plant new ones. It was something she could do. It was concrete. It helped to know that the universe was empty. As was her mother's pain. As was Mercedes herself.

Mercedes framed the severe expression on her face with cascading locks of brown hair. Given to flights of fancy, she was not always dependable or practical. And once Ian dedicated himself to the Three Jewels full-time, her behavior left him agitated. Still, they worked together placing free ads in local newspapers and pasting flyers around the city to promote Roach's upcoming lectures. Occasionally they headed back to his apartment on Roosevelt Island to meditate— always leaving room between him and Mercedes so that nothing physical might happen. Of course sometimes it did, and Kay thought the attraction came more from Mercedes than Ian.*

Christie McNally stirred different feelings in Ian, just as she did for many other people who fell into her orbit.

A year earlier, McNally graduated from New York University, where she studied photography and planned on a career as a photojournalist. She was a tomboyish girl with long, straight brown hair and a captivating and flirtatious smile. She shared a tiny apartment on 13th Street with a roommate and a cat named Max. Like most children of the 1990s, she felt she had missed the major cultural movements of the day. The colorful idealism of the sixties had decayed into the disaffected era of grunge rock. Flannel shirts and callow cynicism replaced the optimism and flowing fabrics.

There had been a string of boyfriends throughout college. Most of them were selected from a small group of friends who seemed to switch partners among themselves rather than search for fresh blood. The last in the line was Ara Babajian, a drummer for an endless succession of bands that almost made it.

The two had great chemistry. They both enjoyed baseball and, like almost everyone in the East Village, experimented with marijuana. She temped at a photo studio while honing her skills as a photographer, but Babajian knew she would be dissatisfied with a nine-to-five life.

They dated for almost a year, when McNally decided to travel to India and Nepal for the first time. She'd been studying yoga and thought that it would be fun to see a new place. Once there, it wasn't long before she found her way to Kopan Monastery about a year be-

---

*In the course of fact-checking this book, Mercedes Bahleda denied that she attended the opening days of the Three Jewels, that she briefly dated Ian Thorson, and that her mother was murdered. She stated that I rely on "poor sources" in my reporting and that what I write is frequently a "complete fabrication." When I showed her newspaper clippings describing her mother's murder, she responded, "No comment."

fore Ian. She was just twenty-two and the teachings had a profound effect on her as she meditated on the nature of emptiness. Like Ian, when she returned to America she sought out a teacher and learned that Michael Roach had begun to give open teachings in Tompkins Square Park to a core group of spiritual students. "They'd talk about Buddhism and then she'd bring it home," said Babajian. When the philosophies didn't mesh with his own path as a musician, the couple drifted apart.

A few months later Roach opened up the Three Jewels. McNally emerged as his star student. When Babajian saw her next, she had five people in tow. "There was a chorus line behind her," he recounted, still baffled almost twenty years later. "I asked her a question and they answered for her." In five minutes they were on their way. Babajian never saw her again.

McNally studied with Roach for about nine months before Ian walked through the doors of the Three Jewels. It was enough time for her to contemplate the most important decision of her life. Would she ask Roach to be more than just her teacher? Would he be her root lama?

The decision entails a sort of spiritual marriage and absolute faith and obedience to one's guru. In an interview in a Buddhist magazine, she described her decision this way:

> Taking a root lama is a very serious [thing]. You have to believe that they're completely infallible and be willing to risk your life for them, offer your life to them, everything. And so, you know, I'm hemming and hawing for like a year to figure out if this . . . I mean I feel called to do it, and I feel a need for a lama, but I didn't want to rush into it. But as soon as I made the commitment, and asked if he would be my root lama, things started happening very very quickly. . . . [I saw] my lama do miraculous things. [And I went] into very interesting meditative states while I was still like wandering around, just spontaneously. Like sitting in a room and all of a sudden seeing every single person as a holy divine being.

In Tibetan Buddhism, taking a root lama creates a sort of indelible connection to a teacher that can't be erased by any sort of worldly action. The vows of obedience work on the spiritual plane and form a connection that persists in all future rebirths. It entails total submission to the will of another person, and complete trust that they will give you the tools you need to progress spiritually. From the moment she took the vows, McNally gave away control of her own life.

Paul Hackett knew that something was strange at the Three Jewels Outreach Center from the moment he walked in the door and saw the pile of shoes in front of the Dalai Lama's photograph. A budding scholar who was working on a master's degree in library sciences at the University of Maryland, he had studied medieval manuscripts and had achieved a mastery of the Tibetan language. He studied Tibetan Buddhism for seven years and was trying to decide whether, at thirty years old, he should shave his head and take the vows to become a monk or meet a woman and settle down. A few years earlier he'd ended what he described as a very stable relationship in favor of Buddhist studies.

More than a decade Roach's junior, Hackett had studied Tibetan at monasteries in Charlottesville, Virginia, and Atlanta. Like most Tibetan Buddhists, Hackett could trace his spiritual lineage backward from one teacher to another all the way to the Buddha. The genealogy of scholarship meant that he was also horizontally related to Roach, sort of like a dharma cousin. His lama, Geshe Jampel Thardo, meditated side by side with Roach's lama, Khen Rinpoche. Together, Thardo and Khen Rinpoche helped found the monastery in New Jersey.

Hackett admired Roach from a distance. Scholars like himself were buzzing with optimism about the Asian Classics Input Project. Text digitalization promised to revolutionize research on Tibetan manuscripts. Much of the Tibetan canon survived only in copies that had been sent as gifts to the great Khan dynasties in Mongolia during a time when Tibet had a powerful standing army.

When the USSR exerted control over Mongolia during World War II, Russian scholars snatched up what texts they could and moved thousands of manuscripts to St. Petersburg. That any texts survived at all was a miracle. Still, their locations posed a problem to scholars around the world who were interested in them. Researchers had to seek permission through arcane bureaucratic channels to mail the cultural treasures across the world. Russian bureaucracy was slow, and not always favorable to outside interests. It was often easier just to hop on a plane to visit the repositories in person. Even then many of the books hadn't been looked at in centuries, and many had rotted inside their silk brocades. Worms cut ruinous paths through the religious treasures and other books simply crumbled from poor care.

In the summer of 1997, Hackett raced up and down the East Coast of the United States in a sun-bleached 1975 VW Beetle, his legs cramped beneath the too-small steering column. He drove from Charlottesville, where he lived with his seventy-year-old lama in a house stuffed with other graduate students. He worked odd jobs and tried to find ways to make money on scholarly projects. When he came to New York the technical director of ACIP, Bob Chilton, asked him to consult on a particularly pesky database problem. Bringing Hackett into the Three Jewels fold would have been a coup for Roach's group.

Hackett sat in on a few lectures and was pleased to see how easily Roach translated complex Tibetan concepts into ordinary English. It was a breath of fresh air compared to the monastic formality that many lamas brought back with them from Asia. He planned to visit Roach in private and speak with him about the dharma.

Later that summer he walked up to Roach's chambers and noticed how bare it was, save only a few books. More surprising was the woman asleep on Roach's bed. Two others lay on the floor. Hackett almost choked. Senior teachers at the monasteries he had seen were never that close to their students, let alone students of the opposite sex. Familiar with the disciplinary tone of Tibetan lamas, Hackett began to yell at the woman to get out. Surely, Roach would be incensed to see a woman in his bed. After all, the man had taken a vow of celibacy. Roach heard the commotion and came out to mollify Hackett, calmly saying, "No, no, it's okay, Paul. I said she could sleep here."

Hackett left with a strange taste in his mouth, but he didn't realize why until a few weeks later when he visited the Three Jewels bookstore again. When he walked through the door to take off his shoes, he paused as his gaze settled on the picture of the Dalai Lama. In Asia, showing the soles of one's shoes to someone else is a sign of disrespect. It would be unthinkable to point them at a teacher, let alone to pile shoes beneath his image. He began to feel the rage curdle in his blood, and thought back to the last time the Dalai Lama was in New York and how people from ACI had been oddly unenthusiastic. An argument broke out in the temple's chamber and one of the students blurted out, "You still think His Holiness is a better teacher than Geshe Michael." The thought left him speechless. Of course he thought the Dalai Lama was a more qualified teacher than Roach. And to disparage His Holiness—the honorific reserved for the Dalai Lama—was tantamount to blasphemy.

Hackett started to kick away the footwear in front of the Dalai Lama's picture. He turned his back on Roach, who was sitting at the front of the room, and prostrated himself in front of the Dalai Lama's picture three times, then walked out of the Three Jewels bookstore for the last time.

The scene didn't make much of a stir among Roach's most devout followers, but a schism was deepening between Roach and Tibetan orthodoxy. Hackett thought Roach might be inventing a religion all his own.

Because Roach's English-language teachings were so easy to understand, his students often felt they didn't need to seek out other Buddhist perspectives. Thus isolated, Roach's students couldn't comprehend the larger struggles between Tibetan theologians. Ian was falling in love with the teachings, and Roach's busy tour schedule gave him an excuse to get back out on the road. Ian helped draft fundraising brochures for the digitization project. He huddled over a computer with a black woman from the Caribbean who had taken monastic vows and changed her name to Ani Pelma. By October he signed up for a three-week retreat with Roach at a meditation center in Redding, Connecticut, called Godstow.

It was Ian's first formal intensive session under Roach's direct supervision, and he borrowed money from his parents to make it happen. A few months later he called on his family again and borrowed from his grandmother to finance a trip to Mongolia. Roach planned to teach to a packed auditorium in Ulaanbaatar, close to the archive that he was in the process of digitalizing. A Mongolian TV channel would cover the event and broadcast it across the plateau to the few Mongolians who had TV reception. Ian would try his hand as a documentarian and tote a small camcorder to record Roach's reception.

Ian traveled cheap by necessity along with Bahleda, McNally, and a handful of Roach's growing retinue. Once there, the stark Mongolian landscape reminded him of jagged hills and barren valleys of Tibet that he'd walked across a year before. It was empty and beautiful and had very few roads. Most people here still rode horses if they planned to get anywhere outside the city. In the city, Ian traveled in small vans and was in charge of carrying everyone's luggage. The video he shot was shaky and its audio muffled by raging winds. In a letter back home to Jan he quipped that he felt he was sometimes more a hindrance to the group than an aid.

Roach lectured on the Diamond Sutra, a treatise that likened enlightenment to the clarity and strength of a diamond. It was the book Roach had studied as a twenty-year-old in India, and which he credited with putting him on the path to enlightenment. The text describes the world in relativistic terms.

Ian's letters home got more personal. Life was impermanent and short, and Jan was old and sick. It was only a matter of time until he passed on. Ian counseled his godfather on the process of death as Tibetans viewed it. He envisioned Jan as a sort of divine being who had come to earth to help Ian make the most of his life. He wrote:

I hope that amidst your flashes of memory you remember your soft gentle capacity for kindness that I have had the fortune to witness from seedling to sapling. Sometimes I wonder why I have been so blessed with people such as you in my life to guard over me with angelic white fingertips. Buddhists would say that I must have done something good in the past. Something immeasurably good, my Jan, something immeasurably sweet.

Ian wanted to be with his godfather when he passed on, but his traveling schedule was making it more difficult to reach Switzerland, where he lived and would likely die.

As he sat on the stoop of a Mongolian monastery, Ian wondered if perhaps the best way to use the short life he had was to become a monk.

He could take the vows, change his name, and devote himself to Michael Roach. He could take Roach as his heart lama, just as Christie had, and devote himself to the search for inner truth.* Perhaps monkhood would give him the direction that he was sorely lacking in his own life.

Ian's writings turned toward the question of evil in the world. If the pen didn't exist on its own (or, in Michael Roach's words, "on its own side"), then nothing did—at least in an ultimate sense. And yet there were deaths all around him. Tibetans were massacred by the Chinese army. He had been held up by cops on his trip around the world. Wars were brewing in Israel and the Middle East. Could all of these things simply be coming from his own mind? Why would he perceive them if they didn't really exist? The teachings had restructured his world. And he meditated on them every day, convincing himself of their truth.

He chewed on the conundrum in a letter to his college friend LaShaun. "I am responsible for lots and lots of evil. Every child murder I hear about on TV: I made them all. The perception of a bad thing can only come from the imprint made in the past of having done something bad."

The counterintuitive thoughts were hard to accept. Though she had a Christian background, LaShaun studied meditation at centers on the West Coast and responded that she too had been having uncanny realizations. Coincidences took on a significance for her that they never had before. Nothing was random. There was a pattern; synchronicity was in the air. She mused that perhaps she too would be interested in becoming a monk. Like Ian, she wrestled with the problems of fully embracing a universe where the only thing that matters is perception. Still, something about Ian's letter struck her oddly. She looked for clarification of

---

* The terms *heart lama* and *root lama* are often used interchangeably in the Tibetan community.

his thoughts. Perhaps it was a path to madness and irresponsibility, not transcendent knowledge.

"Am I correct in my assumptions that to go further in spiritual study and practice would lead further from physical reality? Even as I formulate this question I recognize it as absurd and nonsensical, but perhaps you have the paradox to answer anyway. The simple answer for me may be to just behave appropriate to the reality that I find myself in at the moment," she wrote to him.

The question sat with Ian in his meditations. He wanted desperately to see every moment as intrinsically interconnected and sacred. Meditations brought him bliss, but making that feeling last when he was away from his cushion wasn't always possible. There were still fights with his parents and an ongoing struggle to earn a living.

No, he wrote back to LaShaun in October 1999, he wasn't leaving a connection to the world. If anything, he reasoned, his meditations were bringing him closer to the ultimate clockwork that made the universe run. In a lengthy reply on yellow legal paper, he wrote back:

Our world in the present is made of imprints planted in the past that ripen into a flower. As they wear out it gives the impression of time passing. In a car trees go by, the imprint to see one wears out, then another, and another. It looks like motion. Why do nice moments wear out? Because we don't know how moments are made. If I figured out how to make them I could setup a moment making machine and just let it run: a forever lasting moment? . . . I don't think my spiritual training brings me farther from the physical. Maybe closer. Colors brighten, tastes sharpen. These are all results from nice meditation. It makes the body feel lighter, eventually getting younger and turning into an angel's body. My direct experience only confirms the very beginning of that process, but I can see logically that it happens. Thoughts, ideas, world-view, all have a direct relationship with the physical body. Anger means tense muscles and short breath, so logically, less anger means less tense and ultimately a body of light.

Life was a projection of his own mind. His travels across Asia, his life in a fraternity, and his chance meeting with Roach and Christie

McNally were just karma from past lives playing out. Now that he was beginning to understand how the world really worked, what could he do to make his mind a better place? Could he change his own projections and change the world? Could he find free will?

That question can't be resolved with logic. The answer had to be felt. To be experienced. And the key, Michael Roach taught, was in his own mind. He would unlock the truth with self-discipline.

5.

Programming

Mark my words. There was a time when most of America didn't have Bodhisattva vows. People will interview you about the old days. Mark my words, later you will appreciate it. It's already happened and you don't see it yet. Historically, you were at the beginning.
—Michael Roach, February 2, 2000
At Ian Thorson's Bodhisattva vow initiation

Seeking ego loss is part of the spiritual paradox, for it is the ego itself that seeks ego loss because it believes that not having an ego would be a better state to be in.
—Joel Kramer and Diana Alstad,
The Passionate Mind Revisited

KAY THORSON CUT tomatoes into slivers and sliced oblong chunks off a heavy loaf of bread. She dropped two eggs into boiling water and set the timer so that the yolks wouldn't cook all the way through. Six minutes later she fished out the eggs with a slotted spoon and delicately placed them onto white ceramic stands. She shattered the top of one of the eggs' shell with a metal spoon and then scooped off the broken crown. Steam wafted upward from the gooey interior. Across the table Ian's egg sat uncracked, and she wondered if today was the day he would come down and eat more than just half a stick of butter on toast or a handful of Cheerios.

She was concerned that Ian was acting differently since he'd returned from Mongolia. He refused to leave his childhood bedroom until late in the day. Now he spent much of his time with the door to his room locked, sitting with his legs crossed on a round meditation cushion and his back to the window. If he looked outside, he could see the redbrick Episcopal church, which was one of the few identifiable landmarks of Roosevelt Island. The long wooden bookshelf below his sill overflowed with assorted Buddhist teachings and letter transcripts that he had collected over his time at the Three Jewels. The mess spilled out onto the floor and to the foot of his single bed.

His surroundings didn't seem to matter to him as he turned his attention inward. His heel reached up toward his navel, and his knee rested flat on the floor. It was perfect expression of the full lotus, the meditation pose that both Hindus and Buddhists claim is ideally suited for realizing ultimate truth. His eye twitched beneath his lids as he focused his mind on a picture of Vajrayogini, the goddess of *dakinis*.

"*Om Vajrayogini hum phat svaha,*" he said, exhaling air from his lungs. Like most mantras, the utterance is more a collection of impressions than a logical sentence. It's not exactly Tibetan or Sanskrit. Some claim that the words originate in the neolithic. *Om* is the guttural sound of the universe, the static that has existed since the Big Bang. *Vajrayogini* salutes the goddess by name and *hum* invokes the truth of emptiness. The mantra reaches a crescendo on the word *phat* as it is expelled with a full breath of air almost like a shout. It has no translation except perhaps the sound of a cracking whip. *Phat* adds power to the mantra and concentrates it. Finally, after a short pause, the chant relaxes into *svaha*, a sound that might as well mean "so be it." It can also mean something burning to ashes in a fire. Ian chanted the undulating words in an endless cycle. They washed over the everyday chatter of his mind. Whenever his thoughts wandered elsewhere, he would catch himself and focus again on the words.

The mantra helped him feel the subtle energies that linked his physical body to the ethereal plane. For thousands of years Buddhists, Hindus, and Chinese acupuncturists have mapped out a subtle body that exists in parallel to the inert matter of the body. Where the physical body is made up of blood vessels, muscles, cells, and nerves, the subtle body has its own anatomy. In it, constantly flowing currents of energy called *lung*, or wind, move through riverlike channels called *nadis*. Wheel-like whirlpools called *chakras* circulate the energy currents along a course that mirrors the spinal column. It all travels along a precise route from the sex organs up through the crown of the head. In death, the energy body shucks its links to the flesh and moves onward into a divine realm. As he refined the visions, Ian could feel the winds send electric shivers through his flesh and spirit.

Where a surgeon can operate on the physical body with a knife and sutures, meditators use symbols to define and reform the link between the body's subtle energies and the mind. Vajrayogini is both a goddess and a symbol. If you think of her as a tool, then she can cut a malleable mind as easily as a knife slices skin. It was not the sort of meditation that was supposed to make someone relaxed. It was meant to be powerful. It was tantra.

Ian kept a small *tangka* picture of the goddess Vajrayogini in front of him while he meditated. Roach taught that the quickest way to reach enlightenment was through the goddess's aid. It was a bit of a misnomer: In order to gain her blessings during his meditation, he would have to *become* her. On his own, Ian knew he was a poor vessel for enlightenment. The goddess, on the other hand, was perfect. So if he could visualize her perfectly in his mind, and then think of himself wearing her body, he would prime himself for a profound transformation. The first step was to give up what there was of himself. He begged the goddess for refuge and offered his five senses to her in return. He offered up his sight, his smell, his taste, his touch, and his hearing, hoping she would purify them and allow him a glimpse of the ultimate reality.

Months of training allowed him to bring an image of the goddess to his mind with the ease of a master chess player replaying a game by reading a list of moves in the newspaper. The visions came on like a lucid dream. Vajrayogini stood before him with the body of a sixteen-year-old girl wearing a brilliant garland of severed heads. The heads symbolized his own ignorance. She bled from her vagina, but was also obviously sexually aroused. Her eyes blazed fiery red, and blood dripped from the fangs in her mouth.

Vajrayogini sustains herself on a diet of violence and death. Though she is terrifying to behold, her purpose is good. She eats negative emotions and thoughts, and the act of consumption destroys them forever. In his vision of her, four *dakinis*, fairylike handmaidens with lesser powers, attended to Vajrayogini's every whim and desire. They kill for her and purify the world of ignorance.

When the goddess was crystal clear in his mind, Ian began another simultaneous visualization. He split his mind in the same way that a computer runs a subroutine. He imagined that there was a small Tibetan letter located at the center of his own heart. It was the Sanskrit letter *va,* the root sound for *Vajrayogini.* Bright ruby rays extended outward from it through beyond his field of vision and into the universe. The rays were made of pure love. The letter vibrated with energy. He summoned all of his joy and happiness and projected it through the universe.

Roach had promised that these practices would speed Ian's own transformation into an angel made of pure white light. But now was the most difficult feat of all: full transformation.

He looked at her limbs and then imagined that they were his own. Blood dripped down from the corner of his mouth. He could feel the pert breasts heavy on his chest and the extra limbs extend from joints that he had never sensed before. The symbol of her name burned brightly in his heart. Soon he wore the heavy garland of heads and knew they were also the vanquished seeds of his own ignorance. It was painful and blissful, and at times not completely crystal clear. Eventually the transformation took hold. For a moment he was the goddess. Then he had only one more task to perform. He had to give away all the merit that he had accumulated in his life to the universe.

From inside this new body he looked out to one of his four hands and saw an exquisitely sharp chopping knife. The curved meat cleaver was alive with electricity and power. This was the tool with which he would accomplish his own dissection. Perhaps he grimaced at the weapon as he went to work. He chopped off his hands. He chopped off his feet and cut out his own heart. Thus butchered, he offered up the cutlets and sweetmeats to his voracious *dakini* attendants.

They licked up the blood with their forked tongues, but there was still more of him left over. So he invited demons into the vision and let them feast as well. They arrived one by one with saliva dripping from their hideous mouths. They snacked on the assortment of limbs and tendons. Still, Ian offered himself freely.

Where Ian was, exactly, in this moment was difficult to discern. He was the offering. He was the goddess. He was the *dakinis* and the demons. He was a man sitting on a cushion with his face squinched in focus. This was how he would finally dissolve his ego.

Once the demons had their fill, Ian slowly came back to the world. Layers of reality and imagination peeled back against themselves and he opened his eyes to the white walls of his room. He was on Roosevelt Island again, just across the river from Manhattan and a thirty-minute train ride away from further teachings by his guru. The taut arms of the goddess were gone, replaced by his own spindly limbs. The athletic body that he'd once worn was wasting away since he'd stopped eating regularly. The skin hung loosely on the bone, his knees knobby and his ribs visible from across the room. He smiled at the emaciated form. He was getting lighter and close to becoming an angel.

Kay tried to listen to what was happening behind the closed door, and could hear the cyclical rumbles of his recitations. He had been awake since the sun first sifted its light through the venetian blinds of New York's vertical cityscape. Now it was noon and he hadn't eaten a bite. The egg on the breakfast table was long since cold.

Kay didn't like the new Ian. He wouldn't speak to her until the afternoon, and then only when he was on the way out the door. If she knocked before the appointed hour, he would snap at her. Once, when she was tidying up the house, she wanted to move an old TV console out of the living room and into one of the upstairs bedrooms. It was morning, but the appliance was also much too heavy to handle on her own. So she knocked on his door and asked for help.

The tapping on his door fractured the delicate image he was maintaining. The goddess dematerialized in his mind and all he could hear was his mother's requests. The concentration on his face played into a grimace. "Don't interrupt me unless there's a fire!" he shot at her.

The contrast of Ian's reaction to his goal of compassion for all living things made it hard for Kay to feel respectful of his practice. Something was wrong, and she worried that the more he got involved with Roach, the more she was losing him as her son.

In August, Roach introduced a pink pamphlet with the title "The Book: Make Your Dreams Come True" to his students in New York. Only thirty pages long, "The Book" is perhaps the single most important piece of literature for his students because it prescribes a daily action plan for enlightenment.

In it is a list of 147 vows organized into different categories. Headings include "Refuge Commitments," "Vows of Freedom," "Vows of the Bodhisattva," "Root Downfalls," "The Black and White Deeds," and "The Five Vows of a Lifetime Layperson." The vows themselves come from the Buddhist canon. Roach's innovation was to create a moral accounting system so his followers could audit their spiritual progress.

The pamphlet's instructions state that in order to receive tantric teachings, Roach's followers have to check their vows six times a day for two straight years, pausing every couple of hours to be sure that they were not committing a karmic faux pas. The rules ran from fairly straightforward offenses like adultery and murder to more esoteric, impenetrable, and baffling karmically bad concerns like "Giving up the highest Dharma by discounting the scriptural collections of the way of the self-made Buddhas."*

Intermittently throughout the day, students marked the book with plus (+) or minus (–) signs to indicate whether they kept to the code or faltered on their path. The system was supposed to keep them present and in the moment.

---

*Among these vows is the proscription against idle talk and gossip, which is largely interpreted as a ban on saying anything negative about the community of Buddhists and meditators that they study with. For a journalist, this vow proved repeatedly problematic since many Buddhists—even ones critical of Roach's teachings—worried about breaking sacred vows that tied them into a larger Buddhist tradition. Vows are ranked hierarchically; breaking this *samaya* (commitment to the community) is considered more profound than the vow against lying.

When Ian finally left his room and headed out to the Three Jewels, he always had a copy of "The Book" with him. Old copies became ledgers of his karmic sins. Kay went to his room and flipped through the discarded books and marveled at the hundreds of chicken-scratch check marks. Each one represented a karmic seed. For Kay, the moral record keeping was the last straw. "Roach was taking control of my son's mind. There was no time he wasn't there," she said. It would be her call to action.

While he loomed large in Ian's mind, Roach was concerned with bigger matters. Since the time he founded the Three Jewels in New York, Roach simultaneously raised funds for a very special retreat in the secluded hills of Arizona. He made arrangements to rent a tract of land from a Mormon rancher in the town of St. David, where he would be able to meditate in isolation from the rest of the world. Roach dubbed the collection of yurts Diamond Mountain University even though it was neither accredited nor, strictly speaking, near a mountain. The campus was in a wide valley between distant ranges. Nonetheless, going on retreat was important to Roach and he was very selective about whom he allowed to come along. Only a few chosen adherents could come: Christie McNally; Ani Pelma, a nun who had supervised Ian while they created promotional flyers for the Three Jewels; and two other women—Susan Howler (not her real name) and the nun Trisangma. The goal was more lofty than transforming oneself into a goddess. They would meditate in total silence for three years, three months, and three days and try to gain a direct perception of emptiness. Roach wanted to experience the same twenty minutes of bliss that he had felt when he was making his teacher's tea more than twenty years earlier.

When Roach emerged, he promised he would share his insights and initiate his followers into new tantric teachings. Ian volunteered to help work on the outside of the retreat and ferry food and supplies to the retreatants. It would allow him to remain close to his teacher, even though Roach would not be around to guide his practice in the meantime.

It was an auspicious moment for disappearing. The millennium

was drawing to a close and people everywhere were hoping that the
next epoch would bring change. The retreat would begin in March
2000, and from that date forward, Roach would stay out of the public
eye. The only exception would be three rare and beautiful ceremonies in which he would break his silence and talk to his followers
about what he was learning.

It was called the Great Retreat, and might just be the first of many
such intensive meditation programs in America. In Tibet, countless
masters spent years meditating in remote caves in their own pursuit of
enlightenment. Roach planned to retreat in a climate-controlled yurt.
All he had to do was recruit attendants like Ian to ferry him every
earthly need so he could focus on transforming his mind in solitude.

To fund-raise for the program, Roach planned one last speaking
tour around the world. Ian signed up before he could even figure out
how to pay for the airfare. More than thirty other people signed on to
go with him.

A German woman, named Beatrice Steimer, whom Ian had met
at one of Roach's classes, shared his bed for most of the trip. Steimer
was an artist and a yogini and had the hard edge and formality to her
manner that clings to many Northern Europeans. The qualities
seemed to balance out some of Ian's own restiveness.

In his efforts to ingratiate himself to Roach, Ian took it on himself
to be sure that his guru was comfortable during the journey. The
spicy Indian food did not always agree with his teacher, so Ian dedicated a significant portion of his suitcase to a comfort food diet of
powdered macaroni and cheese, Cheerios, and microwave popcorn.
There were also pretzels, chips, cookies, and sweets that might keep
up Roach's spirits in a time of need.

The first stop was a small storefront called the Himalayan Buddhist Meditation Centre. Situated in Kathmandu's tourist ghetto of
Thamel, the meditation center gave teeming masses of European
backpackers easy access to a quick Buddhist teaching. In the morning
they could pay a few Nepali rupees for a lecture on emptiness before
chowing down on Buffalo cheeseburgers nearby or catching a Nepali
band covering American rock songs at a bar.

The center was a key recruiting base for the FPMT—the Foundation for the Preservation of the Mahayan Tradition, which ran Kopan Monastery, where both Ian Thorson and Christie McNally first studied Tibetan Buddhism—and an ideal spot for Roach to raise funds for the Great Retreat. He lectured on the nature of karmic seeds and the possibility of accessing ultimate reality through meditation. Back in St. David, Arizona, set in the craggy valleys between the Dragoon and Chiricahua mountains, dozens of students assembled retreat yurts for Roach and the other retreatants. Roach spoke to the audience about what sorts of miracles might come out of a thousand days of silent meditation alone. There would be strict rules. None of the retreatants would so much as see another person in that time. The very stillness of their surroundings might allow them to crack the veil of emptiness. The FPMT tacitly allowed Roach to raise funds for the project, even though their policy was not to let guest teachers gather money for things not directly affiliated with the foundation.

After five days of lectures, the troupe went overland on a poorly maintained highway from the Nepali capital to the holy city of Bodh Gaya. It was the reverse of a journey that Ian had made several years earlier. The two-day trip took them south across the border at Birganj and into India in time to hear the Dalai Lama give nine days of teachings to usher in the new millennium.

While Bodh Gaya symbolizes the ultimate attainment of enlightenment for most Buddhists, the rest of the state of Bihar is one of the most corrupt and violent states in India. Still controlled by feudal landlords called *thakurs*, Bihar never achieved its dream of democracy. Armed bandits prowl the roadways, looking for a chance to rob unsuspecting travelers. Still, thousands came to hear the Dalai Lama's teachings. Roach made arrangements to capitalize on the crowds when he set up his own public lectures a few days later at a local FPMT center called the Root Institute.

Foreigners who had trouble listening to stilted translations of the Dalai Lama's speech over transistor radios would be keen to listen to an American geshe explain Buddhist concepts in plain English. In a way, scheduling his own teaching right after the Dalai Lama's lectures may have been a subtle signal that Roach was on par with the supreme leader of the Tibetan tradition. The Root's walled compound is just outside the town. Ian unloaded the geshe's bags from the back of a rented white Tata Sumo SUV and placed them in his teacher's private quarters. Roach's retinue booked the majority of the rest of the rooms.

Every day the ragtag group of Roach's Western Buddhists made their way to the Bodhi Tree—which is thought to be a direct descendant of the original tree where the Buddha sat when he achieved enlightenment—and sat on small rugs and listened to the Dalai Lama lecture in Tibetan. When the Dalai Lama finished speaking, Roach's followers invited anyone they could to hear Roach lecture on the Diamond Cutter Sutra.

It was hard not to notice that McNally and Roach had become inseparable. No matter where he went, McNally was right behind her teacher, carrying a black laptop bag with a bulky premillennial computer inside. Ostensibly, they worked together translating complex Tibetan scriptures. She had become his sergeant at arms, strictly enforcing the rules he set with a hard look. Occasionally she'd pull someone aside for a stern reprimand. She was tough, and their closeness could be disconcerting. When Roach visited the bathroom downstairs, McNally stood outside the door. Her syntax had begun to change too. The Valley girl cadence morphed into a patois of English and Tibetan. One student remarked that it seemed like she was trying to impersonate Yoda. When Roach was tired of teaching, sometimes the twenty-six-year-old McNally would fill in and lecture on emptiness.

Anthony A. Simmons, a balding director of the Root Institute who ran countless meditation programs for the FPMT, kept a wary eye on Roach's comings and goings. Roach wore the robes of a Geluk monk, the same order as the Dalai Lama, which was also the same lineage as the founders of the FPMT. As such, Simmons expected that Roach would adhere to the traditional rules for monks, which had been passed down since the time of the Buddha. Chief among these rules are proscriptions to dress appropriately and refrain from sexual conduct.

Yet every morning he heard that Christie McNally left her geshe's quarters and snuck back to her own room. Simmons presumed they were sharing a bed. For lay Buddhists, sex wasn't a problem, but Simmons worried what it would mean when a rising star among American Buddhists violated his lifetime vow of celibacy.

Simmons didn't know exactly what to make of Roach, but he was wary of how an outsider might judge the FPMT for embracing an iconoclast monk. Simmons didn't have the authority to do more than lodge a report of the possible infractions with people who were close to Lama Zopa Rinpoche, the founder of the FPMT.

Rumors spread that Roach took liberties with the teachings of the Buddha—or that McNally might end up spending more time alone with her teacher than Roach was advertising on the retreat. Ian, for his part, looked on in awe at his teacher, and was sure that what other people called strange behavior should be viewed as another lesson in the dharma.

Also on the trip was Matthew Remski, a young yoga practitioner from Toronto who had attended more than two hundred of Roach's lectures. Remski watched McNally and Roach's secretive canoodling but didn't worry that it might violate old-fashioned traditions. Roach was building a new Buddhism, and perhaps the religion needed new rules. Remski had shared countless meals with Ian on the cross-India trip and was equally enamored of Roach's philosophy. They ate thin dal together at the group hostel, but Remski couldn't help feeling alienated from Ian. They talked philosophy, but Ian was uniquely uncurious about subjects outside the ultimate truth he was seeking. For Remski, Ian's tousled hair and unfocused, trancelike eyes indicated some sort of underlying neurological problem. During lectures, Ian inadvertently shook with apparent ecstasy—his legs jumping and his eyes rolling into the back of his head. It wasn't an unusual performance in and of itself; indeed, the front row of Roach's lectures was often full of ecstatic people. In a letter he posted online,* Remski wrote that Ian displayed "severe and rattling *kriyas*—spontaneous bursts of internal energy that jagged up his spine, snapped his head back sharply, and made him gasp or hiccup or yelp or bark." Most students took the movements as a sign of openness to kundalini—the libidinal energy that yogis teach is the essence of creativity. He was either joining his subtle body to his physical one, or something was going very wrong in Ian's mind.

The tour continued from Bodh Gaya to the beaches and tourist hotels of Goa. From there it turned southward to Roach's lineage monastery of Sera Mey in the Indian state of Karnataka. Perhaps aware of brewing controversy, Roach closely watched the movements of his students. He issued a written directive in mixed capital letters forbidding any of the people in his entourage to talk with the monks of Sera Mey without direct supervision. They weren't even allowed to walk around the compound on their own.

The Tibetan refugee settlement outside of Mysore, where Sera Mey is located, is considered a restricted area by the Indian government, and Western travelers typically need a special permit to travel inside. Yet the warning applied to any student of Roach's, no matter if they had arranged their own permits or not. The message was clear: If they came to Sera Mey, they would keep to themselves or risk being kicked out of Roach's entourage, possibly forever. "Be good bodhisattvas and BE CONSIDERATE of the others to come in the future by following the policy exactly." It began with an appeal to compassion, striking home its point with a threat. "If any student violates the above policy, Geshe Michael will inform the local police and local Indian federal authorities that this person is not part of our group, in order not to jeopardize the other students."

Ian had been to Sera Mey on his world trip before. Indeed, he met

*Matthew Remski's Internet epistle on the website *Elephant Journal* titled "Psychosis, Stabbing, Secrecy & Death at Neo-Buddhist University in Arizona" is one of the most revealing portraits of the history of Diamond Mountain ever written. A member of the group for several years, he brings an insider's knowledge to the sect along with the dispassionate analysis of an expert critic. The letter galvanized a movement of people around the world who had fallen out with Michael Roach, and structured the first coherent critique of the events that eventually took place in Arizona.

Roach through a recommendation from the monastery's abbot and even brought back bronze statues and incense to Howell, New Jersey, as an introduction. Still, there were no exceptions to the rule. Ian shuttled back and forth to the talks in a white tourist bus every day. He made no mention of the policy in his own letters home, but carefully folded the warning with his notes from the time. After twelve days of teachings, he boarded a flight back to New York, where he intended to tell his mother that he was ready to make one of the most important commitments of his life. He wanted to become a Bodhisattva and was ready to take vows that would publicly commit himself to the path of enlightenment by taking Roach as his heart lama.

Only six days would pass between the moment when Ian's plane touched down in New York and when he would report to a small auditorium in the East Village to confirm his Bodhisattva status. When Kay heard the news, she was awash with emotions, not the least of which was relief. "At least he wasn't going to be a monk," she recalls now with bittersweet sorrow. Bodhisattva vows meant that although he would be committed to Roach for life, at least he wouldn't wear robes and shave his head too.

Even so, it might be only a momentary reprieve. She and her husband began working on a plan to extract her son from Roach's sway.

She knew Ian wouldn't listen to her if she said it to him directly, so she needed a plan that would appeal to his intellect. She would need evidence. She would have to become a detective to look for cracks in the skein of enlightenment. When she arrived at the small auditorium she covered up a miniature tape recorder in her lap with a white legal pad and set the machine spinning.

She conspicuously doodled Roach's face on the legal pad so that Christie and Mercedes wouldn't notice the recorder and confiscate it. The two women walked up and down the aisles of the chamber to be sure that everyone took the ceremony with the correct disposition. Though it wasn't a tantric initiation, the meeting was still secret. And Kay reasoned that the transcript she wrote up would be useful to anyone whom she enlisted to help get Ian away from the group.

Roach sat on a raised stage and welcomed the prospective vow takers and invited anyone in the audience who was inspired to take vows along with them. It was supposed to be a joyous occasion, yet the audience sat in solemn silence.

"Once you take these vows you do not take them again, okay? These vows last until you give them back or you die. You can banish them, but you can't get rid of them unless you formally return them or die," he said.

The permanence of the commitment made one initiate's voice crack when he asked what would happen if he broke one of the smaller ones.

Roach smiled and decided to answer with a familiar metaphor. He reached into his robes and pulled out his favorite instructive tool: a black pen. On cue, an eight-year-old girl skipped over to the podium and got down on all fours and began barking like a dog. The audience laughed as she put up her hands like paws and began panting. She reached for the chew toy. "Are you okay?" he asked, beaming during the moment of levity.

"If you keep these vows, your karma will force you to look at this pen differently." Intentions are everything, and vows that are supposed to set lifelong patterns are extremely powerful.

"It is impossible that an act of honesty could lead to any kind of problem. It's impossible. That's the first law of karma. You cannot ever lose anything from keeping your vows. You have to understand that. If you are honest and then somebody hurts you, there is no cause and effect there. The only cause and effect is that if you keep your vows you must get wholly wonderful results. And if you break them you can't get a good result," he explained.

"If you break it, even unknowingly, you plant a seed in your mind to see yourself as a dog in a future life." Breaking other, higher vows, such as talking bad about a dharma teacher, could earn a student a stint in Buddhist hell where demons might roast the vow breaker on a spit for hundreds of consecutive lives until the karma gets cleaned.

Roach looked out at the initiates with a stern face. Then he motioned them to rise. Ian stood up in his best buttoned-down shirt in the middle of the group. On cue, they bent at the knees and prostrated themselves before the geshe as one. It was time to mark this moment as a permanent commitment to their lama.

"We'll do it in Tibetan, because you take it more seriously if it's in a foreign language. When I'm done I'll snap my fingers and then you've taken your vows. This energy just entered your mind stream."

Roach lifted his fingers to his mouth, and the audience was silent as a grave. He began to read a long passage in Tibetan. Ian knelt with his hands pressed; his eyes were closed as he focused on the vibrato of Roach's voice.

Vows poured off Roach's tongue like liquid. When the stream of Tibetan stopped, he snapped his fingers and Ian said his own name out loud.

The tape recorder in Kay's lap whirred to a stop and clicked off.

6.

Deprogramming

For the most part [participants in esoteric cults] are at a loss to explain what happened to them. Many, however, describe it in one graphic, almost visible term. "Something just snapped inside me," they report or "I just snapped"—as if their awareness were a piece of brittle plastic or a drawn-out rubber band. And, indeed, this is often the impression of those who are closest to them: their parents, spouses, friends and colleagues. To these observers, it appears as if the individual's entire personality has "snapped," that there is a new person inside the old one, someone completely different and unrecognizable.
—Flo Conway and Jim Siegelman, *Snapping*

Secrecy is endemic to both the structure and the metaphysics of Roach's organization. Buddhist knowledge was secret. His relationship with McNally was secret. Whether or not it involved intercourse was secret. The instructions for rituals were secret. The nature of his realizations was secret. The locations and identities of many of his teachers were secret. Tantric practices were secret. In the absence of physical coercion, secrecy was the key currency of Roach's power.
—Matthew Remski, *Elephant Journal*

KAY THORSON SAT in her son's room and worked her mouth around a word salad of Buddhist terms—*Bodhisattva, samsara, samadhi, bodhichitta, emptiness, lama, rinpoche*—that seemed to require an advanced degree to decipher. Now that vows bound Ian to Michael Roach, she would have to act quickly or she might lose her son forever.

When Ian left the house for a meeting at the Three Jewels, Kay and her husband, Tom, scoured the boxes of notes and materials that he had left pell-mell across his room. To them it looked less like Ian had been meditating and more like he had been brainwashed. The Bodhisattva vows that Kay recorded required him to scrupulously account for every thought and movement he made. Roach's routines kept Ian too busy to question why he was doing it. As she sifted through the pile, one heavily underlined leaflet stuck out to her. It was a list of daily instructions seeming to offer not only the promise of good things to come but threats if Ian didn't stay in line.

Her eyes lingered on one command in particular: "You must recite it every day, Thrice in the day, thrice at night. If you fail, a fault of practice becomes a serious offense. . . . I bow first to the lotus feet of the One who Holds the Diamond, the Lord, My Glorious Lama. . . . The refuge objects before me completely dissolve into white, red and blue light then merge into me. My body and wealth, I offer without reservation."

At least Roach couldn't enforce the code directly. He was several thousand miles away just at the beginning of a silent retreat that would keep him out of circulation for three years. His control over Ian was more about habits now. Ian listened to tapes and did coursework in his free time, and had begun to talk to his parents about his desire to head out to Arizona and sign on to become a caretaker on the Diamond Mountain land. There Ian would cook food for Roach and the other retreatants and make sure they could focus entirely on their spiritual progress without having to worry about the stresses of the outside world.

Kay and Tom's diagnosis: Their son was in a cult. Michael Roach was a cult leader.

They called a psychologist in New York for advice and the doctor suggested that the best way to get someone out of a cult was to enlist the aid of people who'd given over everything to a religious group and still managed to extricate themselves. He gave the Thorsons the names of two cult deprogrammers.

In the 1980s, Patrick Ryan and Joe Kelly dreamed of levitation.

They practiced floating on the sprawling campus of domes and ochre classrooms of the Maharishi University of Management in the middle of the Iowa flatlands and in Transcendental Meditation (or TM) centers in Philadelphia. Back then, Ryan and Kelly sat on meditation cushions and asked the Hindu god Krishna for his divine blessing. The oldest text in yoga, Patanjali's *Yoga Sutras*, devotes an entire chapter to pseudomagical powers called *siddhis*. The ancient text says that truly devoted students can learn to levitate, to turn their bodies invisible, or even possess another person's body. TM teachers promised that their students would one day stay afloat and hover in the middle of the room. To outside eyes the technique was almost comical. They sat in full lotus posture and bent forward until they coiled at their waists like cobras. With their legs still crossed beneath them, they sprang upward and managed a small hop in the air. During the brief moment of apogee—when the grip of the earth overcame the force of their jump—they could almost imagine they were weightless. Inevitably the moment didn't last and they crashed back down to the matted floor.

Ryan and Kelly practiced for almost a decade as they watched the university grow rich on hefty initiation and program fees. When the miraculous abilities never materialized, the two grew cynical and joined a class action lawsuit against TM. They held picket signs outside of new-student initiations and warned prospective students against the spiritual path that TM was selling. The Maharishi declared the protesters apostates to the cause. The litigants countered that in all the years of its existence, Transcendental Meditation had failed to produce even one successful instance of antigravity.

Margaret Singer, a Harvard psychologist who developed clinical theories on mind control, testified at their trial and declared that Transcendental Meditation fit the classic criteria for a cult. The World Plan Executive Council, the controlling body for TM, hired a battalion of lawyers to defend the case. Rather than drag the process on for years, Ryan and Kelly settled out of court and reaped a portion of the money they had spent on TM classes.

While the two men failed to win a victory in open court, the lawsuit showed them that they were not the only people who believed they had been taken advantage of in the name of enlightenment.

They began attending conferences of disaffected spiritual seekers, and delved into the academic research on cults. Soon people began asking them to help with friends and family members who had been sucked into alleged cults. There were Christians who believed that the Apocalypse was near, Buddhists hell-bent on Nirvana, and New Agers who espoused a mishmash of free-flowing energy theology. No matter the ideology, the stories fit a pattern. Adepts fell for the promises of a charismatic leader and then withdrew from their families and friends. As insiders, Ryan and Kelly understood what it meant to be consumed by divine thoughts. By 1990, they began working their cases as exit counselors.

They weren't the first. The field of deprogramming grew in the United States after a series of violent episodes drew attention to apocalyptic ideology. In the 1960s the countercultural revolution helped usher in a strange tide of new religious movements. Some were imported from foreign lands, others homegrown. Most were considered harmless until, in 1969, members of the Manson Family committed a string of murders in California in the name of an apocalyptic vision. Followers of Charles Manson killed actress Sharon Tate, the pregnant wife of the movie director Roman Polanski. They cut out her unborn fetus and painted the words *Helter Skelter* on the wall. Manson became the poster child for a cult leader who could transform ordinary people into psychopaths. Just nine years later, 909 followers of Jim Jones ingested cyanide at his Peoples Temple in Guyana. Just before they took their own lives, Jones's followers assassinated American congressman Leo Ryan, who was there on a fact-finding mission into the group's activities.

While the vast majority of fringe religious groups can only be considered benign by comparison to Jones and Manson, people who found their loved ones suddenly sucked into an unfamiliar group worried about worst-case scenarios. At first, the field of deprogramming employed drastic tactics that seemed to match the potential hysteria of cults themselves. Ted Patrick, a pioneering deprogrammer, kidnapped cult members and held them against their will until he was convinced he had undone the religious psychological conditioning. He put his clients under psychological duress, yelling at them and challenging every statement they made. Eventually the person's mind gave way and, Patrick claimed, they simply snapped back to their former selves as if someone had pressed the reset button. He earned the name "black lightning" from his victims. The tactics backfired on Patrick when judges reasoned that the new methods amounted to unlawful imprisonment before they sentenced him to several stints in jail.

Kelly and Ryan were cut from a different cloth than Patrick. Preferring the term *intervention* over *deprogramming*, they aimed to reason with their clients instead of shocking their system. Once they could engage Ian in conversation, they figured he would empathize with their own stories and it would help him recognize the parallels to his own situation. Kelly and Ryan's results are less dramatic than Patrick's but fare better under legal scrutiny.

When Kay and Tom called the exit counselors, Kelly and Ryan estimated that the process might take a year and would cost a total of $35,000. So Ian's parents put 10 percent down and started mailing the counselors audiotapes, notes, and videos by Roach. Together they would have to create a plan that would convince Ian to leave the group of his own free will.

"There is no cookie-cutter approach. We're not going to show up in our deprogramming capes like superheroes and just fix it," said Joe Kelly more than ten years after the original intervention. While the initial sit-down might go quickly, the family needed to prepare and understand Ian's thoughts as much as possible to be ready for any intellectual way out that he might throw up. "We want the dialogue to be respectful and the family to understand the appeal of the group to the person. Ian was investing his life into this. It is important that when you are interfering with an adult's life that they need to feel respected."

Ian's family wanted the intervention to happen as quickly as possible, but the counselors cautioned that it would likely take six months or more to make the proper arrangements. The key was to show Ian that despite whatever realizations he had achieved, his actions still left a real-world footprint.

To do that, Kay and Tom would have to bring all of Ian's family and friends together and show him what he meant to them. So as Ian planned new meditation retreats and kept careful accounting of the vows, Kay sent e-mails and letters to every friend who wasn't affiliated with Diamond Mountain whom Ian knew. She contacted Saul Kato and Mike Oristian from the fraternity at Stanford and sent letters and reading lists to his high school girlfriend, Fernanda Hannah, and to Ian's grandparents. They set a date for the summer, when Kay expected Ian would be the most relaxed.

For six months Ian had no inkling of the plot except that life for him seemed easier. The family backed off and allowed him to get comfortable. Ian used the permissive atmosphere to persuade his parents to let him use the two-story saltbox house they owned in East Hampton for his own private meditation retreat. In happier times the family used it as a base of operations to surf early-morning waves on nearby beaches, so ordinarily the house was stuffed with surfboards and beach paraphernalia. However, in the last few years, the family's finances were stretched perilously thin. The cost of the intervention, not to mention private tuition for two children at Stanford, put them in a precarious position. When an investment that Tom made went south, they had been forced to put the house on the market. In the meantime it was vacant, and Ian asked for the keys.

As spring took hold, five people from New York—all men—took over the house. They plastered over the windows with construction paper and cleared away furniture. They stocked the cabinets and refrigerator with simple heavy foods that wouldn't take much time to prepare. Ian brought a box of white cassette tapes of Roach's talks and then they sealed themselves off from the outside world. It was a perfect cocoon of silence. Ian's eyes were glassy when he emerged weeks later. Kay bit her lip and swore to herself that it would all turn around by the summer.

New York was humid and miserable in the sweltering month of

July. The sun cooked the Atlantic Ocean, sending an intolerable wave of muggy air across the city. Humid breezes slowed down and came to a standstill as they festered in the long concrete slats the streets form between high-rises. It was on such a day on Roosevelt Island that Kay and Tom invited Ian home to dinner to meet with a few religion experts they thought Ian might appreciate. When he arrived from business at the Three Jewels, Ian greeted Kelly and Ryan and sat down on the couch next to his sister. His grandmother was also there; when his parents couldn't afford the rest of the money for the session, she cut the remainder of the check.

Everyone in the room came prepared except Ian. They'd studied lectures that Michael Roach had given and read deeply into the growing number of books on cult mentality and mind control. "We were hoping that he would just snap out of it," remembered Kay, who watched her son with nervous eyes.

Ian sat in front of them with unkempt hair and listened to his family's worries. They said he had been withdrawing from them, that his devotion to Buddhism had sapped energy away from his professional ambitions. They worried that he was too thin. Ian listened at first and fielded their inquiries like a tennis player volleying balls over a net. He loved all of them. How could he not? He consoled them, told them not to worry about his future: One day he would be a dharma teacher and make a living giving lessons to a flock of his own students.

Joe Kelly decided to prod points of contention that Ian might have with the group. There had to be a way to insert a wedge between the student and his lama. "Why is it that Geshe Michael only selects the most attractive women for his special initiations?" Everyone knew that Roach and McNally were close. They might even be living together on this retreat in the desert. What qualified her for special teachings and not Ian? What could McNally see in a man more than twenty years her senior? Why did Roach preach celibacy for his followers when he got to play by a different set of rules?

Ian's face flushed at the insinuation. Kay and his grandmother asked him why he couldn't see a contradiction. Why he couldn't admit that perhaps Roach's motives weren't always perfectly pure. Ian was trapped, and he knew it. He choked down angry words and seemed lost for a moment. Then, without an explanation, he sprang to his feet and shot across the room to a sliding glass window that overlooked the old stone church. He yanked at the aluminum frame, and the window gaped open. Then he jumped two stories down to the courtyard below. His sister and father went to the window and watched as he rounded the corner at full tilt before he disappeared. Kay remained on the couch. "I'd seen him do it before." She shrugged with the patience of a mother used to eccentricities. Next time they would have to lock a window.

Ian returned on his own later in the evening, but the sudden flight set the pattern for the next three weeks of talks. His family could push him, but if they went too far, he'd look for escape. So when they moved the venue of the intervention to a rented house in Montauk, it was partially with an eye toward not letting him get away so easily.

It was also far from the Three Jewels. "We were near the beach and the water. The places that had always been healing and rejuvenating for the family," said Kay. In the mornings they let Ian stick to his meditation routines as long as, when he emerged, he promised to stay and talk with the family.

Ian had spent almost a month at the beach when it seemed that he was beginning to think about what life might be like outside the group.

He tried to run away only one more time. They were on the way back from the beach with surfboards strapped to the roof of their yellow station wagon, and someone brought up Roach. Ian got flustered. When they pulled up to a light, Ian opened his door and began running in the other direction in just bare feet and board shorts. Kay swung the heavy automobile around and followed him. There was nowhere else to go, so Ian reluctantly got back in.

The whole experience bewildered Ian. Never having thought of the dharma as cultic, he was shocked that his family thought he had fallen so far astray. He sent off a letter to Amber Moore, who had once been a familiar face at the Three Jewels but who moved to Arizona to attend to the Great Retreat. She was in charge of cooking

Roach's food and ferrying supplies to and from the retreat yurts. It was the job Ian had originally volunteered for.

It is so weird my mom thinks that I'm in a cult. So does my dad, and so does my sister. They talk to me in soft voices like I'm a mental patient and tell me that the ACI people aren't ill-intentioned, just misguided. Talk about the emptiness of the LAMA! . . . I tend to think that if the whole world was not madly in love with my lama at least they would respect him and see him as a positive influence. It is a bit difficult to see parents as real beings really holding this viewpoint. . . . Beatrice calls and my mother refuses to give the phone to her and erases her message. It's a lot like living in some weird concentration camp where things are controlled. I'm beginning to feel very much adrift. My former places of refuge are crumbling one by one, leaving only my lama as untouched and perfect. Is there anywhere to go besides near my lama?

Ian's high school sweetheart, Fernanda Hannah, was staying in the city. When Kay felt that the counselors weren't making progress anymore, she reached out and requested that Fernanda hop on a jitney bus to the Hamptons. Fernanda had read everything that Kay had sent her and couldn't help but worry about how Ian had changed.

Ian hoped he would find an ally in her. They went off alone together and he confided to her that he was being forced to make a choice between his family and the spiritual progress he felt he was making. They chatted about what he was learning and then he dozed off as she stroked his hair. She was happy they were connecting and let him rest until she began to feel the tingles of her leg falling asleep. She tried to move him and worked her hand under his head. It was light. Way too light. Since he'd stopped eating in favor of spiritual progress, she discovered, his muscles had wasted away.

"I lifted his head with just one finger he was so light. He had once been this beautiful and athletic surfer boy; it didn't make sense why he would do this," she said.

Later that evening they stayed in his room together and she reminded him of the constant letters and phone calls they had sent each

other through the years and during his travels. They had been each
other's first sexual partner, and she offered herself to him again,
thinking that perhaps a physical connection might help him see the
beauty of the world. "Ian had always been comfortable with sex," she
said. She touched him, but he refused and rolled to the side of the bed.
He needed that energy for his meditations, he said. She was hurt. And
rejected. The next morning, Ian popped a cassette tape of one of
Geshe Michael's speeches into the stereo. They listened together.

In the recording, Michael Roach's voice warbled out of the speakers as he pontificated on the necessity of detachment. Fernanda remembers the tape vividly. "He [Roach] said that you could only
become your own person and really know yourself if you kill your
parents." She paused and then said it again in her high melodious
voice. "Kill your parents. Kill your parents. Kill your parents. It was a
metaphor. Cutting your umbilical cord and connection to the past,
but he kept repeating 'kill them.' It was scary," she said.

The message may have been a reference to an old Buddhist alle-
gorical question: "What should you do if you meet the Buddha on the
path to enlightenment?" The correct answer being: "You should kill
the Buddha." Ultimately, every student needs to find their own way
to Nirvana and eventually even the Buddha becomes an obstacle.

Rejecting Fernanda may also have been a practical matter. Since
traveling to India, Ian had deepened his ties to Beatrice Steimer, a
woman who freely embraced her mystical side. Kay had tried to keep
Beatrice away. She screened Beatrice's calls.

Beatrice hadn't always been as enamored of the rigors of Buddhism as Ian had. She favored a more egalitarian approach to spirituality. She spurned authority figures and preferred a direct connection
to the divine. A deck of tarot cards could be a gateway to the spirit
world; open flames might offer her a glimpse of the universal. If Beatrice had known there was an intervention brewing, she would have
warned Ian away, but now that she was on the outside, she pleaded
with Kay to let her come. As August drew near, Kay agreed.

Ian's sister, Alexandra, saw Beatrice as a wild card. On one hand
she could speak Ian's language. On the other, she might present an

opportunity for Ian to think more positively about Roach. "Part of the problem was that she actually liked my brother, not the group. I felt like she was doing these meditations only to be with him. She would dabble with different Buddhist groups and not be affected by it because she's a space cadet. The problem with my brother was he goes deep into things. I did seven years of Latin, he might have done more. We have discipline. Beatrice's lack of discipline protected her."

When Beatrice finally arrived, Fernanda was still at the summer cottage. In a few hours she realized that Ian's lack of interest in her had less to do with his staying spiritually pure than it did with having moved on. "They were all over each other," she remembered with a sigh. "It was the worst thing that could happen." Beatrice and Ian meditated together, bonding on the possibility of ultimate truth. Fernanda imagined Beatrice casting her sideways victory glances.

As the summer waned, it was unclear whether Beatrice ruined the intervention or saved it. Caught between his family and his heart lama, Ian lacked any fresh options. Beatrice offered a sort of middle way where he might be able to focus his intensity on building a steady relationship. Yes, he might still be searching for truth in meditation, but they wouldn't have to return to Roach's orbit. It was a compromise that his family thought just might work.

When the family boarded up the house in Montauk and returned home, Ian wrote a letter to LaShaun. "I just brought an old girlfriend and close friend of ten years into the same room as my current love. I could not help but give her more attention. Fernanda was so upset. I'm no good around more than one close friend at a time. I get nervous about who I am supposed to treat, and how," he wrote. His family bought him a ticket to Florida, where he would spend a week with his father's parents. He didn't yet know that another exit counselor—a Dr. Langone—was waiting for him there.

Emotions tugged him in different directions. He wanted independence from his parents and friends, but he didn't want to lose them either. More than anything else, though, he wanted an adult love, not the remnants of a love begun in adolescence.

I don't know why anyone would treat someone else as anything less than an angel. I treated my Buddhist friends special, and took my family for granted. But I did it to such a typically Ian intensity that they thought I went crazy. Responsibility. I really don't have a choice but to grow. I have to leave that little kid body behind and it feels right and good to do it. I think I have found a direction that I want to grow towards. So, to make the jump. That is what is next.

Before he boarded the plane, Ian talked to his father about different possible futures. Perhaps graduate school. Studying Buddhism might fulfill his intellectual side, let him get deep into religious philosophy, and also maintain some perspective. It was an appealing thought to both father and son. They looked through graduate catalogues for religious studies programs around the country. It was all so cordial until what could have been a promising conversation descended into an argument because Ian felt his father was trying to control his life. Ian ended up boarding the plane angry.

When he next spoke to Beatrice, they decided that they needed to move somewhere neutral. Neither Arizona nor New York would do. Maybe he should come with her to Germany and try making his own way out of everyone's reach. He would find the stability that his family said was missing. He could start a career on his own terms. He didn't need Roach. He didn't need to be an angel. He didn't need anyone but her.

Within a year, Beatrice was pregnant.

7.

Diamond Theosophy

Never before had I encountered a truth I was willing to lie for.
　　　　　　—Stephen Batchelor, *Confession of a Buddhist Atheist*

Asia had been read and, at least historically speaking, misread many times over.
　　　　　　—Catherine Albanese, *A Republic of Mind and Spirit*

KAY THORSON LAID a sheet of plain brown paper on her kitchen table and aligned two books by Michael Roach in the center so that the corners squared perfectly. That morning she pillaged the box of Ian's notes and removed samples of his ACI homework as well as vocabulary lists of Tibetan words. She folded the documents around a compact disk that contained a talk Roach gave on the nature of emptiness. The echo of the monk's voice in her mind sent a cold shiver down her spine. The paper wrapped easily around the bundle and she completed the package with precise corners that resembled the sheets of a hospital bed. When it all was tight and well contained, and she was sure they wouldn't break free, she flipped the package over and inked in an address at the University of Michigan.

The intervention bought Kay some time. Ian was on a flight to Germany with his girlfriend and far from anyone at Three Jewels. Still, she couldn't shake the feeling that it would all fall apart again. What would happen when Roach came out of retreat and began teaching? Would Ian fall back into his fold? She had to be prepared and wanted to have ammunition that would speak to Ian's intellect.

The package was destined for a professor of Buddhist and Tibetan studies named Donald Lopez. Two years earlier, Lopez wrote a book titled *Prisoners of Shangri-La* that undermined some of the fantasies Westerners tell about the Tibetan Plateau. Kay hoped that Lopez might be able to tell her if the teachings Ian learned were authentic. Lopez wrote back almost immediately.

> *To claim that these doctrines and definitions mean the same thing in 21st century New York that they meant in old Lhasa is not something that scholarship can decide, but is rather a matter of religious faith. This is not something that I could decide for your son. However I can say that the definitions that your son is memorizing are not an eternal wisdom, but are the products of a very vibrant and contentious history. There is a vast range of interpretation of Buddhist doctrine, both within and among the sects of Tibetan Buddhism. Indeed, the actual content of the doctrines is sometimes less interesting than the history of their formation.*
> —Donald Lopez, September 27, 2000

As Kay searched for the authentic message of the Buddha, she began unpacking a convoluted history of religious interpretation. In the case of Tibet, it all started when a single monk strapped a few tattered manuscripts to his back and carried the germ of Buddhism across the Himalayas to Tibet in the fifth century. The Sanskrit text was meant to be an offering of peace, but the king of Tibet was too interested in waging endless military campaigns against his Chinese neighbors to pay the books much heed. The documents moldered untranslated on a shelf for more than a century until the great monarch Sontsang Gampo came across them in his archives and ordered his scholars to translate a few pages to see if they held anything worthwhile. It was merely curiosity on his part, but the sweetness of the Buddha's words spoke to him from across the ages. He yearned for more and his spark of interest spread into a conflagration.

In the following thousand years, Tibet sent countless emissaries into India to study in monasteries, translate sacred texts into Tibetan, and bring the knowledge back home. Perhaps the vast, desolate, and picturesque landscape lent itself to meditation. Whatever the reason, the thirst for Buddhism consumed the country in a way that it never had in India. They filled palaces and libraries with books; each text was carefully printed on loose pages and then wrapped in a silk brocade and shelved. Over the centuries, books became a type of currency for the elite that was more important than money or property. The texts contained sacred knowledge—a sort of divine umbilical cord to the Buddha himself.

Pilgrims from the countryside who could not read showed their respect for the dharma by walking in wide circles around the book repositories. They hoped that merely being near the sacred texts would earn them a better rebirth. Those who were brave enough to endure the arduous journey to India and return with esoteric teachings became heroes on the order of Davy Crockett and Lewis and Clark in the American West.

For the poorly equipped traveler, the Himalayas are a near-impenetrable barrier of icy peaks and abysmal chasms. At any moment the mountains might come to life and break off in a deadly avalanche—entombing the unlucky in a frozen hell. Once they cleared that particular danger, pilgrims had to descend more than two vertical miles along bandit-ridden roads where the cold mountains leveled out into foothills. Farther along in their journey they trekked across the blistering hot and humid Gangetic Plain. Here they found disease, incessant heat, and tiger-infested jungles.

Those lucky enough to penetrate the natural obstacles did not find the holy cities hospitable. Indian monks who ran Buddhism's oldest monasteries had little more than a passing curiosity for foreigners. The prospective pilgrims had to literally beg the headmasters of universities to let them begin their studies; only then could they attempt to assimilate ancient Pali and Sanskrit books. The language presented its own barrier. First the monk had to learn Sanskrit to even begin the project, and it could take years to struggle through each book's for-

eign vocabulary. Where there were no adequate translations, scholars had to invent new words in Tibetan to explain esoteric concepts.
Translators copied the Indian archives by hand and wrote their versions on the fallen fronds of palm trees.

Most pilgrims died on the journey. Others chose to stay and continue their studies on their own. Yet, those rare few who did make it
back to their homeland reaped rewards befitting royalty. Students
flocked to their teachings, and scribes sent copies of the translations
to the farthest reaches of the Tibetan Empire. If they wanted to,
translators could hold sway on the political and economic affairs of
the entire country by bending the dharma to their own uses.*

Translators were more than just a conduit between India and Tibet; they were active participants in the flavor of Buddhism that came
home with them. By the time Tibetans took an interest in the words
of the Buddha, the literary tradition for Buddhism in India was already mature and various schools of thought competed for promi-
nence. While some teachings were said to come directly from the
mouth of the Buddha, others originated much later from famous
teachers who had their own versions of enlightenment. For the trip
to be worth it, translators sought out the teachings that their countrymen had never heard before: the rarer, the better. Sutras that
taught ethical imperatives might be suitable for a wide audience, but
the translators learned that tantric texts earned prestige back home.

Modern scholars who have studied the original manuscripts were
unsurprised to learn that the translations that endured the legions of
miles on monks' backs were not always true to the source material.†
Occasionally, texts that turned up in Tibet were little more than the
insights of a monk from his travels, but the books nonetheless mas-
queraded as sacred texts from an ancient source. Ronald Davidson, a

---

*The scholar Ronald Davidson writes in *Tibetan Renaissance* that translators became some of the
most powerful political players in Tibet—unifying vastly different regions of the country. "While
local lords were geographically restricted in their authority, translators could claim all of Tibet as
their range in their propagation of the Dharma."
†The problem is hardly limited to the Tibetan Plateau. The field of hermeneutics is entirely devoted
to bridging the gray area between idiosyncratic meanings. Countless gallons of ink have been
spilled on moving the Bible from one language to another. In the end, it is almost impossible to
prevent drift in a text as it takes on new forms in new contexts.

professor in New York who spent much of his lifetime poring over translated books from medieval Tibet, found that in many cases the tantric scholars borrowed freely from non-Buddhist sources, including the wide array of Indian mystics, magicians, and yogis they met on their travels. As translators hurried back home with increasingly outlandish literature, Buddhism there took a turn toward the exotic. Stories of *siddhas*, enlightened masters with magical powers, spread freely.

The problem of authenticity was as relevant in medieval Tibet as it is now that Tibetan Buddhism has gone global. Does authenticity mean an indisputable connection to an ancient source of wisdom? Or can something be authentic even if it is ephemeral and experiential? Perhaps the questions are best thought of as a tension between what has stood the test of time and what makes someone feel a connection to the spiritual ideal. Either way, the religious scriptures worked their way across medieval Tibet like a geological force. Over more than a millennium, Buddhism changed Tibetans' relationships to the landscape and crafted a symbolic spiritual world. As the traditions splintered and broke apart, Tibetan Buddhism spawned generations of contentious debates and controversial leaders.

In the 1300s, a portly monk named Dolpopa donned the pointy red hat of the Sakyas and started a debate on the nature of enlightenment that still roils through religious life today. Dolpopa spent his life traveling mostly through southern Tibet and Nepal, meeting with reclusive monks and scouring their libraries. In 1333, he consecrated the largest stupa in Tibet in a green valley between rolling hills where he liked to lecture from its alabaster ledge. Until then, most Buddhist scholars held the view that everything in the universe was constantly changing—even enlightenment itself. Dolpopa considered this hogwash. Yes, lots of things were in flux, but there were fundamental rules about how the universe operated that were true across all time and space.

Dolpopa taught that there is a pure ultimate reality that is as solid as bedrock. What is more, a kernel of experience flows through from one life to another. He used the Hindu word *atman* to describe what

a Christian might call the soul. Gaining enlightenment meant understanding the true clockwork that makes the universe work. Any person who achieved enlightenment would effectively become infallible
because they could understand the true karmic consequences of any
action.

Fierce debate erupted throughout the Himalayas. Dolpopa's fame
grew and he gave teachings to thousands of students about the nature of time and reality from inside his humble valley. Dusty pilgrims
and layfolk laid out garlands and butter sculptures in his honor. The
institutions he left behind generated wealth on the order of kings,
and for a time, Tibet's political and military center revolved around
the south of Tibet.

The pendulum began to swing in the other direction six years
before Dolpopa's death in 1361, when a remarkable child was born in
a valley known for its robust onion production. His name was Je
Tsongkhapa. Whispers circulated that the child was the reincarnation of Atisha, one of the first people to bring Buddhist texts to Tibet.
By the age of twenty-four, Je Tsongkhapa was ordained a Sakya monk
in the same lineage as Dolpopa. All of Tibet anticipated that he would
be one of the most important teachers of the age.

Tsongkhapa devoted himself wholeheartedly to the study of monastic vows and the importance of a rigorous social order. He became
known as a great reformer, and his most vehement objections were
aimed at dismantling Dolpopa's legacy. Tsongkhapa argued that there
was no such thing as an ultimate reality; even the notion of emptiness
was in itself empty of an inherent meaning. No human could ever
expect to attain final communion with divinity. Buddhism, according
to Tsongkhapa, was about the process of discovery, not about attaining a final goal. This shift meant that no person could claim to have a
realization closer to ultimate truth than another person's. Everyone
was potentially fallible, and a monk's worth ultimately boiled down to
how well he adhered to the earthly rules that the Buddha left to his
followers. In effect, Tsongkhapa asked his followers to have faith in
enduring institutions instead of mystical insights.

Tsongkhapa founded what soon became the most important and

powerful sect of Tibetan Buddhism. Dubbed the Geluks, they set
themselves apart from other monastics by wearing yellow hats that
curved forward over their foreheads. They built the Potala, a
thousand-room palace in Lhasa, and installed the Dalai Lama as its
ruler. In time Lhasa grew into the most powerful city in Tibet. The
Geluks raised an army, and then fiercely suppressed Dolpopa's writings.*

The popular image of Tibet is that it is a sort of meditative paradise full of peace-loving monastics and contemplative debate. However, war was no foreigner to the high Himalayas. Throughout
history Tibetan armies marched between monasteries and brutally
put down insurrections and upstart warlords.

One famous encounter started when the king of Tsang, a patron
of the Karma Kagyu—another Tibetan Buddhist line of thought—
challenged the authority of the 5th Dalai Lama and began sacking
Geluk monasteries in the south of Tibet in 1642. The Dalai Lama sent
emissaries to Gushri Khan, a descendant of Genghis who ruled Mongolia, to ask for his aid. The Khan was loyal to the Geluks, so he and
his Mongolian cavalry descended on Tibet like a hot wind. They cut
through the Tsang armies and put thousands of monks to the sword.
When the Khan came to Lhasa, he gave homage to the Dalai Lama
and rode back to Mongolia with the treasures from sacked monasteries. Armed conflict broke out at least seven more times before the
Chinese invaded in 1959.

Time has a way of favoring institutions over the charisma of leaders, and Dolpopa's charm has been mostly relegated to the dustbin of
Buddhist history. His name is now most often remembered only in
reference to how Tsongkhapa defeated him on the debate field—
something that, historically, couldn't have occurred. But the tension
between Dolpopa and Tsongkhapa is mirrored in every faith that
seeks to justify its own existence. Which is more important? Striving
for a direct communion with the divine or building something on

---

*Some scholars suggest that Dolpopa's philosophy didn't fail because of Tsongkhapa's rhetorical
powers as much as because of geopolitical realities of the time. As the Geluks gained power, they
raised powerful armies to enforce their philosophy at the edge of a knife as frequently as they did
on the debate ground.

earth? And if a person can experience God, is he above worldly criticism?

An important test to that tension came thirty-six years after Tsongkhapa passed away. Born in what is present-day Bhutan, a cherubic lama named Drukpa Kunley became known for teaching the dharma through the tip of his penis. The sexual aspect of tantric teachings was nothing new to Tibet, nor was it particularly uncommon to hear stories about lamas who misused their position to take advantage of their students. Kunley, however, took his tantra to the extreme. He was a self-described madman who had no respect for the traditions laid down by institutions. Instead, he drank endless quantities of alcohol, wrote bawdy poetry, and impregnated both layfolk and nuns. As a skillful orator, he convinced high lamas to reclusive virgins that, by surrendering to his will, they would be taken down the path to enlightenment. His poems satirized Buddhist scripture. In a typical example, he poked fun at the way Buddhists are said to take refuge in the Buddha. Instead of surrendering themselves to the dharma, Kunley insisted that they salute his penis.

> *I take refuge in an old man's chastened penis, withered at the root,*
>   *fallen like a dead tree;*
> *I take refuge in an old woman's flaccid vagina, collapsed, impenetrable,*
>   *and sponge-like;*
> *I take refuge in the virile young tiger's Thunderbolt, rising proudly,*
>   *indifferent to death;*
> *I take refuge in the maiden's Lotus, filling her with rolling bliss waves,*
>   *releasing her from shame and inhibition.*

That Kunley wasn't pilloried, drawn and quartered, or torn apart by a mob is a testament to his ability to sway people to his view. He became a folk hero and his enduring legacy mostly stemmed from his ability to perform miracles. Since he couldn't ground his authority in an institution, he proved that he had progressed along a spiritual path by performing *siddhis*.

In one famous event, Kunley urinated off the roof of a palace in front of a crowd. Before the yellow stream of urine splashed onto the ground, he sucked the piss back up through his penis, presumably with an impish smile on his face. Perhaps, then, it was fitting that he left a mark at the places he visited, lectured, and seduced women. In present-day Bhutan countless houses and monasteries bear his symbol on their walls. In these paintings a giant erect phallus and scrotum showers seminal fluid from the top of its engorged purple head. The ejaculate sometimes drips grotesquely down the wall in homage to the idea that sexual unions can be a conduit to enlightenment. People who are unprepared for such an image in a temple often gasp at the sight.

Kunley, and other saints like him, were adepts of what is commonly referred to in modern times as crazy wisdom. In these sorts of teachings, people give in to their passions and tear taboos asunder in order to make a profound point. Georg Feuerstein, a Buddhist scholar and follower of one of Kunley's modern successors, wrote that "in the eyes of the world [Kunley] is a radical, an anarchist or eccentric—a lunatic. His very existence calls into question the established order. Living as he does . . . he has no need for any self-limitation. His entire life is a towering symbol, a constant demonstration, of the fact that the limitations the 'usual man' presumes are merely neurotic strategies to introduce a semblance of stability and orderliness into the incessant flux of events that constitutes phenomenal existence."

Perhaps Kunley also benefited from a Buddhist concept known as *upaya*, which in English gets translated as "skillful means." While the teachings of the Buddha seem to fit a logical order, the precepts have to function inside a world of politics, war, deceit, and injustice, and it isn't always expedient to follow all of the vows perfectly. So a realized person may take certain liberties with Buddhist rules, as long as they are applied "skillfully." Kunley could get away with catcalling at princesses and daughters of warlords because he convinced them that he broke the rules for their own benefit. Since Kunley had achieved the highest state of enlightenment, they would just have to trust that he knew what was better for them.

Tibetan Buddhism succumbed to the same weaknesses and

abuses of power that afflict just about every other religion at one point or another when mystical experiences take precedence over tradition. Replete with madmen, reformers, charlatans, conflict, and fundamentalism, there never was just one undifferentiated stream of Buddhist teachings, but many that reflected particular historical moments. It's not strange that debates that happened in medieval Tibet continue to pop up in modern-day depictions of the Himalayas.

There are many potential starting points to the West's fascination with Tibet. Ancient traders moved spices, cloth, and ideas across the seas and over the Silk Road. The tales that came back from the East bore the hallmarks of myth and exaggeration just as they had when the first Tibetan translators returned from India. Medieval travelogues relied heavily on fantastical tales with only the slightest peppering of factual reporting. As Europeans looked east they envisioned lands populated by manticores, dragons, and men who, in lieu of heads, had their eyes and mouths inscribed into their chests. The most absurd notions dissipated with time, but the East retained a mystique of undiscovered secrets.

In the eighteenth and nineteenth centuries, European colonies spread out across the globe. The puppet governments they installed were effective at extracting massive amounts of wealth from the farthest reaches of the planet and depositing the proceeds in Western banks. The process was violent, racist, and ultimately a failure, but it was also the first time in history that the majority of the world was shunted into a single economic and philosophical vision. Europeans liked to think they had a "civilizing" effect on the planet. When they weren't busy building railroads and waging war in India, some British, German, Russian, and American missionaries and bureaucrats also combed through sacred Asian texts to develop more compelling arguments that would convert people to Christianity. The Bible made its way into indigenous languages and, as part of the exchange, religious texts from around the world came to Europe.

By the mid-1800s, a German named Max Müller became the most

noted early scholar of Indo-European languages.* He translated classic Sanskrit texts that he found in the East India Company's archives and introduced the *Rig Veda* and the *Upanishads* for Western consumption. The academic interest helped legitimize the writings of orientalist authors like Rudyard Kipling, whose books conjured an India populated with snake charmers, fearsome animals, and mystical swamis.

As the British cinched their control of the continent away from local rulers, they were surprised to learn that few people there actually displayed magical powers. Still, the prevailing assumption was that these magicians were simply rare commodities. Somewhere in Asia, there must be yogis practicing in ca   who could perform inexplicable feats. After Europeans had circled the globe on tall ships and decimated native populations in North and South America, there was really only one place Westerners hadn't yet penetrated.

Even as late as 1900, only a handful of Westerners had ever made it into Tibet. Its borders were guarded by a weak army, but the Himalayas were significant enough to keep all but the most intrepid explorers at bay. With the rest of the world explored, Tibet was the last place left to cast fantasies.

At the same time that Kipling was writing from his post in India, America was undergoing its own spiritual reformation in the wake of the Civil War. The unprecedented casualties on the battlefield made many people question the existence of a Christian god. Why, after all, would a beneficent creator allow so much suffering in the world? During a period known as the Great Awakening, the devout sought out direct personal experiences with God instead of using the church

---

*The Indo-European language family consists of 429 identifiable languages that share a common root. While there are various theories for how languages have spread across the world, one of the most widely held assumptions is that the first Indo-Aryan speakers came from what is now Armenia around 4000 BC. These people, known as Aryans, domesticated horses early and were able to spread their language in an area that stretched from Spain to Eastern India. According to the "Aryan invasion hypothesis," this is why German and Sanskrit share a common grammatical structure. This linguistic theory became important during the rise of Nazism to support the notion of a master race. In India, there is a popular notion that the reason people in the north of the country tend to have lighter skin than people in the south is that they descend from Aryan stock. When the Aryans came, they supposedly conquered the dark-skinned indigenous people who spoke Dravidian languages. Whatever the truth is of this prehistoric warfare, these early scholarly endeavors to uncover historical languages often cloak the current racial politics of the day. See Edward Said's *Orientalism* for a more complete discussion.

as a go-between. The more esoterically minded also looked for faith outside of a Western context.

The most influential person to capitalize on the West's newfound interest in Asian religions was a Russian mystic named Madame Helena Blavatsky. When she was just seventeen she married a forty-four-year-old man but quickly turned sour on the union. So she stole a horse and fled west into Europe. Over the course of the next ten years she found acceptance in the budding spiritualist community, billing herself as a psychic and spirit medium. She traveled to Egypt and immersed herself in the shadows of the pyramids. There she hunched over a crystal ball and communed with occult powers in a perfect pantomime of how we like to think fortune-tellers look. In 1873 she moved to New York, claiming to have been initiated into secret tantric practices by Buddhist masters in Asia. The word *tantra* was still new to the American audience and it tantalized their nascent beliefs in occult powers.

At one of her séances in Vermont, Madame Blavatsky met a prominent lawyer and Civil War hero named Colonel Henry Steel Olcott. They joined forces and founded the Theosophical Society, whose mission statement said it was formed "to promote the study of the world's religions and sciences, and to vindicate the importance of old Asiatic literature; and to investigate the hidden mysteries of nature and the physical and spiritual powers latent in man."

Theosophy held that every religion accessed a sort of universal spiritual truth. Whether you call it god, divinity, or a universal soul, Blavatsky and Olcott believed it was possible to interact with what Kant called the noumenal realm. By rigorously (and in many cases unrigorously) comparing different beliefs in different religions, they hoped to uncover the truth of God in the same way that archaeologists uncover ancient civilizations. They would compare ancient Indian scrolls to Mayan Prophecies and Jewish Kabbalah and hope to find a hidden kernel of wisdom that ran through all of the writings.

The blend of rationalism and occultism proved immensely popular among the American and European literati. In 1879 the pair moved to a compound in Madras (now Chennai), India, and raised funds to translate as many Indian and Tibetan texts as possible. Scholars and spiritual seekers of the day found that Theosophists offered the most stable base to finance logistical support for their work.

Drawing upon her earlier experiences as a spirit medium, Blavatsky channeled a group of divine philosophers that she called the Mahatmas, or great souls, who lived in remote caves on the Himalayan Plateau. Every morning the Mahatmas sent her handwritten notes and left them in a wicker basket in her bedroom.

The hundreds of letters she received over the years eventually ended up in a manifesto called *The Secret Doctrine*. In its first week in print, it sold more than a thousand copies and went on to be a bestseller for decades. Outside of spiritualist circles, academics and religious authorities often rolled their eyes at her pronouncements. After all, it was far more likely that she placed the Mahatmas' letters by her bedstand when no one was looking.

Even so, the Theosophical Society's efforts to deliver Asian religious texts for mainstream consumption was hugely influential. The historian Catherine Albanese wrote, "The 'secret doctrine' of Asia would provide the vocabulary and grammar for a generic metaphysical discourse. In it Asian historical particularity was effaced, and the universalizing potential of concepts like reincarnation, karma, and subtle bodies was amplified many times over. Arguably, the general American metaphysical project of the late twentieth and twenty-first centuries would continue to sound themes and enact Asias that originated in the Blavatsky opus."

In other words, Blavatsky's reimagined Asia spoke to America's malaise with the modern world. It formed the grammar of the New Age movement that we take for granted today. Theosophists financed the first translations of the *Tibetan Book of the Dead*, the *Yoga Sutras of Patanjali*, and various gnostic gospels as well as popular translations of the *Bhagavad Gita*, the *Upanishads*, and the *Tao Te Ching*.

As with Tibetan translators who brought books from India in the medieval period, Theosophical translators imbued their works with an agenda that thrives on sensational experiences. By 1920, Blavatsky was dead, but the Theosophical Society had grown to more than forty-five thousand members worldwide. Their influence continues to be almost impossible to factor out of any project that references the spiritual traditions of Asia.

By 1904 the Himalayas were not the barrier they once were. As a reminder that the British were not concerned foremost with Indian literature, Lt. Colonel Francis Younghusband invaded Tibet with a force of nearly three thousand seasoned fighters. Tibet tried to defend its borders with soldiers armed only with muzzle-loading muskets and protection amulets. The British responded with automatic fire.

The campaign followed a familiar colonial pattern of massacre and pacification that would be as familiar to the Apache and the Zulu as it was to the fallen fighters on the Himalayan Plateau. In the first encounter, more than seven hundred Tibetans fell in just four minutes. One lieutenant in charge of a battery of Maxim guns wrote, "I got so sick of the slaughter that I ceased fire, though the general's order was to make as big a bag as possible. I hope I shall never again have to shoot down men walking away." A *Daily Mail* correspondent who was one of the few British actually wounded in the battle wrote, "The impossible had happened. Prayers, charms and mantras, and the holiest of their holy men had failed them. They walked with bowed heads, as if they had been disillusioned in their gods." By July of that year, the British entered Lhasa and forced Tibet to pay a large indemnity, and accept a British trade mission.

For more than two hundred years, Lhasa had practiced a strict policy of isolationism. Whenever a foreigner crossed into its borders Tibetan authorities politely escorted them back across the Himalayas. The British occupation ended that. After Younghusband's lopsided victory, erstwhile travelers could apply directly to the Crown for the rare, but technically possible, entry permit.

In practice, however, the British tried to keep Tibet isolated because it served as an ideal buffer between their government in New Delhi and the Chinese's constant westward expansion. The few people stationed in Lhasa were career bureaucrats who were uninterested in doing much more than intergovernmental relations. They denied hundreds of applications for travel until, in 1937, an Arizona native named Theos Bernard used diplomatic magic and a large amount of cash and received an entry permit. He became the first American to set foot in Tibet.

Bernard's uncle was Pierre Bernard, better known as Oom the Omnipotent, who claimed to be a tantric yogi. Oom was wildly popular and managed to open a chain of tantra clinics in Cleveland, Philadelphia, Chicago, and Manhattan. Oom is probably best known for linking *tantra*—a word that refers to secret sacred teachings—to sexual mystical experiences. In a familiar twist of gurus gone bad, in 1910, police arrested Oom after two teenage girls accused him of kidnapping them and allegedly brainwashing them into sexual bondage.

Theos Bernard tried to distance himself from his uncle's reputation but still seemed to have studied in the same school of thought. He hoped to find texts in Tibet that expounded on the sexual side of tantric teachings. If he could find them, then as their custodian he would be in a position to become an influential teacher. From there he planned to make a fortune selling his story on a lecture tour.

Bernard spent about six months traveling across Tibet, taking thousands of photographs and hundreds of feet of film with an early movie camera. He toured the Potala Palace and hired important lamas to perform elaborate ceremonies that he could record. When he returned to the West a year later, he appeared in public wearing the crimson robes and yellow hat of a Geluk monk. Despite his very brief stay in Lhasa, he declared to the *Daily Mail*, "I am the first White Lama—the first Westerner ever to live as priest in a Tibetan Monastery, the first man from the outside world to be initiated into Buddhists' mysteries hidden even from many native lamas themselves."

He toured across America for the next ten years, claiming that the Dalai Lama recognized him as a reincarnation of the eighth-century saint Padmasambhava, who is arguably the most important teacher in the entire religious history of Tibet. A fawning American public believed Bernard. His portrait graced the front cover of *Family Circle*, which was then one of the largest-circulation magazines in the world. He established the now-defunct American Institute of Yoga and published his bestselling book, *Penthouse of the Gods*, about his experiences.

A few years later, Columbia University awarded him its very first PhD in religious studies for his work on Tibetan tantra and Indian yoga. Over time, profits from the speaking tour eventually leveled out, and with his fortunes dwindling, Theos returned to India in 1947 with the intention of finding more lost books.

Giving little heed to the politics of the day, he began his search in Northern India when the country was in the throes of an independence struggle. After World War II, Britain teetered on insolvency, and British holdings in Asia no longer turned a profit. At the same time, a massively popular nonviolent movement led by Mahatma Gandhi undermined the premise that India needed to be "civilized" by British colonialism. So the British decided to relinquish control of India.

The British planned to break the colony into two different countries along religious lines. India would be mostly Hindu, and Pakistan mostly Muslim. As members of the two communities scrambled across the border to their respective new territories, the entire region erupted into a conflagration of violence. More than a million people died and sword-wielding militias massacred entire trainloads of refugees as they attempted to flee across the new border. Bernard got caught up in the conflict while poking around old Buddhist monasteries. Most likely someone shot and killed him somewhere in the Himalayan foothills. His body was never found.

Bernard is something of a model for many of the Western gurus and monks who have since come back from Tibet with claims of spiritual specialness. As he beamed with authenticity from beneath his robes, there were very few people in America who knew enough about Tibet to raise objections against his claims of enlightenment. On the other hand, without people like Bernard and Blavatsky, Eastern religions might never have gained a place in the popular imagination. Military campaigns like those led by Younghusband might have extinguished Tibetan Buddhism as a primitive, heathen, or merely irrelevant belief if scholars in Europe hadn't gotten caught up in its romantic notions.

The People's Liberation Army invaded Tibet and forced the Dalai Lama and a retinue of hundreds of monks into exile in India. Pictures of the exodus appeared in newspapers around the world and elicited waves of sympathy. The 1959 flight marked the end of any real hope for Tibetan autonomy, but also forced the Dalai Lama's impoverished government to look for support from Western allies. Unlike other marginalized ethnic communities under China's iron fist, Tibetans had one commodity that endeared them to the international community: their spirituality. And because of that, soon there would be a lot more enlightened Westerners.

At the same time that Tibetan Buddhism was gaining a foothold among Western audiences who sought transcendent wisdom, another philosophical stream called New Thought brewed in the heartland. At the turn of the twentieth century, anything seemed possible in America. The hardships of the Civil War faded from living memory and new inventions like electricity and the automobile heightened productivity and allowed people to see the world in ways they never had before. Night became day at the flip of an electric switch. Advances in vaccines and antibiotics cured diseases that were once death sentences. Along with that wave of optimism came the great fortunes of American entrepreneurs. Tycoons like Andrew Carnegie, Henry Ford, John Rockefeller, and F. W. Woolworth came up from poverty and established vast fortunes. Their rise solidified the reality of the American Dream for the millions who thought they might emulate a fraction of the same success.

New Thought created a spiritual framework to explain earthly success. It came in the form of a recipe and spawned the entire genre of self-help books. Also termed the "law of attraction" as early as 1906, its core belief was that thoughts become things. In 1908, Andrew Carnegie met a young journalist named Napoleon Hill and asked him to interview the richest people in America to learn their secrets to generating wealth. The project took him almost twenty years, but in 1934, he published *Think and Grow Rich,* which quickly became one of the bestselling books of all time.* Hill wrote that the

---

*By Hill's death in 1970, *Think and Grow Rich* had sold fifteen million copies. Its success has since been dwarfed by *The Secret,* which has reportedly sold fifty-six million copies worldwide, with approximately the same philosophy.

most successful people on earth followed a simple secret: They visualize their own success and cultivate their emotions to feel as if they had already achieved their goals. According to his theory, wishes act like magnets in the spiritual ether and can attract real-world riches. Alternately, someone who is perpetually concerned with failure attracts only failure. Thoughts of sickness attract sickness.*

New Thought lent American optimism a sort of mystical quality. It argued that the mind is a force of nature in the same way that gravity is. Thoughts can make a person rich, cure disease, reduce the harm of aging, and achieve any other imaginable goal. Every few years New Thought resurfaces—most recently in the television film and then internationally bestselling book *The Secret*. Millions of people who read *The Secret* created collages of their desires out of magazines—pasting pictures of luxury cars, future lovers, happiness, and health on poster boards. These so-called vision boards are meditation tools that help people visualize their goals. In that way, they're similar to Tibetan *tangka* paintings.

When Michael Roach entered the Great Retreat with Christie McNally, the slow course of history had already mapped out the spiritual terrain for his teachings. Generations of enlightenment seekers, and self-help literature, made his version of Tibetan Buddhism palatable—plausible, even.

---

*In this sense, New Thought seems to derive from Calvinists, who believed that God's favor would play out in the lives of people predestined for Heaven. The resulting divine hierarchy seems to suggest that people who have earthly success are chosen by God.

I have stayed together
In the great retreat, in the proper way,
With a Lady, who is an emanation
Of the Angel of Diamond, a Messenger;
And I've undertaken the hardships needed
To try to complete the two stages
Of the secret teachings.
So too nowadays
To help to trigger
The final transformation into
The Diamond Sow herself,
I wear my hair
As the Angel Herself does,
And her bracelet
And other accouterments
Together with my robes

—Michael Roach
An excerpt from "Letter to My Lamas"

8.

Skillful Means

Retreat is supposed to be a sacred space; a place where you can leave the outside world completely and go into a totally new and divine realm.
— Lama Christie McNally, April 2012

MONGOLIAN YURTS PROTRUDED out of the Arizona desert like a tent camp from prehistory, or perhaps a colony on Mars. The sun cooked the parched plain between the Chiricahua and Dragoon mountain ranges, and the uplift of hot air brewed billowing storms of dust. The gray half domes undulated in the unrelenting wind but managed to protect their inhabitants well enough from the desert's brutality. The jagged spines of two ranges marked the horizon, though they were still far enough away that Diamond Mountain University was a mountain in name only. This was flat land.

At dusk and dawn, boarlike creatures called javelinas prowled across the dry washes and rooted through the scrub brush; their sensitive snouts could detect anything edible hundreds of yards away. It wasn't long before the sharp-tusked animals located the garbage piles that the spiritual pioneers left untended.

Cow pastures flanked the pitted dirt road to the site. Mormon ranchers would sometimes chase wayward cattle past the fence wire despite the warning that the retreat was technically off-limits to outsiders. The proscription against trespassing on the inaugural site for Michael Roach's university might have held more weight if the ranchers had remembered that their own ancestors settled the land as a haven against religious persecution.

In a little-known footnote to American history, a small troupe of Mormon refugees fled from Missouri and founded the nearby town of St. David in 1832. At the time, the United States was searching for a coherent spiritual identity and was easily threatened by radical religious groups.

Wherever they went after the prophet Joseph Smith found sacred golden tablets from the angel Moroni in Palmyra, New York, the Mormons met resistance among locals. When they settled in Missouri the governor of the state raised an armed militia to push the Latter-Day Saints from the state. He threatened to exterminate the ones who didn't leave. One high priest, a man named David Patten, tried to stand and fight, rather than flee from unjust violence. Patten claimed to be able to heal the sick and dying. His fiery sermons recounted a personal meeting with Cain, the fallen son of Adam, who he said had stayed on earth to destroy the souls of men. Patten said he could hear the voice of God himself, and he believed that the approaching militia was little more than the vanguard of demonic forces led by a corrupt government. Armed with muzzle-loading muskets and squirrel guns, he led a small Mormon force against the militia and met them in a small skirmish called the Battle of Crooked River.

The Mormons were sorely outmatched. In the first minutes of the engagement, militiamen shot Patten through the bowels. He died in pain hours later and took with him the Mormon will to resist. The survivors fled to the Arizona frontier, where they hoped they could practice their religion freely. They named the town St. David in Patten's honor.

Roach, like Patten, believed that he had a direct connection to the divine. For him the pursuit of spiritual insight was more important than any social convention. It could transcend life itself. Indeed, was it really that strange that he wanted to use solitude to find a divine message?

Jesus fasted in the desert for forty days and forty nights before he heard God. So did Mohammed. The earliest writings out of Asia mention yogis spending years in caves contemplating Nirvana. Christian and Jewish monastics observe vows of silent reverie. Thousands, if not tens of thousands, of Tibetan monks do the same. The Great Retreat in St. David was special if only because it was the first Buddhist retreat of its kind on American soil. Roach had prepared for it since he began teaching tantra to a select few students in 1995.

At twenty years old, Roach had had a vision that he was on the cusp of enlightenment, and he wanted to get there as soon as possible. Throughout his life he'd seen what he called angels in the guise of the people around him. Their secret purpose exposed the hidden machinery of the universe. To any doubters, he could cite his success in the diamond business as proof that his method worked. Karma explained his ability to generate real-world riches. His followers buzzed with electric excitement. If Roach could transform into a Bodhisattva, then he could help them on the path too. Yet, out of his thousands of followers, only the most fit were permitted to accompany him on his journey. All women. All attractive. All in their twenties and thirties.

The retreatants spoke of themselves in the vein of the great explorers of history. While Neil Armstrong walked on the moon and Christopher Columbus sailed to the New World, these five retreatants were traveling to the remote corners of their own psyches. Loved ones might be nearby; they could come as caretakers and prepare food or write them occasional letters, but they weren't allowed in or to see what Roach or the others were doing. It would be affection only at a distance. For Christie McNally, going into retreat like this was a little like preparing for dying. She tried to make her parents understand. They never did. Yet she said that the sense of history and of urgency drove her forward.

It was a belief that other people could get behind and even dedicate their lives to. Amber Moore was still a teenager when she agreed to take on the responsibility of being the primary caretaker to the retreatants. Unlike most people at Diamond Mountain, who came to Buddhism later in life, Moore was raised in the tradition by her mother, who took ordination vows to be a nun while Moore was still a child. Despite her age, by the time Moore came to Diamond Mountain, she had spent almost the same amount of time absorbing Buddhist ideas as Michael Roach had. Where Roach followed the tradition of the Dalai Lama, the Gelukpas,* Moore's mother was Karma Kagyu, a lineage of Tibetan Buddhism that emphasizes mystical experiences. She was close enough with Ian Thorson to trade letters with him even while he negotiated his way through the intervention.

Before the retreat started, Amber met Roach in New York and asked him to officiate her vow of celibacy. The sexual atmosphere at the ACI courses was hard to deny, but Moore felt that sex caused too much distraction.

They scheduled the vows in advance, and Moore arranged to meet Roach in the East Village. He wasn't there when she showed up, so she searched him out upstairs. As she creaked up the flight of steps, she found Roach and McNally in a saccharine embrace. They massaged each other's hands and gazed deeply into each other's eyes. "It was quite a contrast to what I was about to do," she remembered. They chatted for a few minutes and then Roach came downstairs with McNally and witnessed her vow in front of a statue of the Buddha. For Moore the vow made particular sense because for the next three years she would have very few opportunities to do anything other than care for the five retreatants in Arizona. A boyfriend would divert her energies from the tasks at hand. As far as she was concerned, what Roach did was his own business.

A few weeks later she moved into her own yurt on a desert plain thick with mesquite brush. She didn't observe the same vows of silence as the retreatants, but most of the time she felt much more isolated. At night the stars shone like millions of jewels out of a black sky. Every day had a long routine: She picked up healthy foods at the store in town, then she boiled and chopped it all into a hearty meal that she could serve her wards. Every night, she collapsed on her mat-

---

*There are four major schools of Tibetan Buddhism: the Geluk, Nyingma, Sakya, and Karma Kagyu. At various times each of these rival lineages came to control the religious sentiments of vast swaths of Tibet. Occasionally different factions went to war against one another to eliminate rival philosophies. By the end of the sixteenth century the Gelukpas dominated Central Tibet out of the capital of Lhasa. Each order maintains different requirements for its followers and clergy. Gelukpas make their monks disrobe if they want to do tantric sexual practices. The Karma Kagyu are much more liberal.

tress and listened to the distant howling of coyotes. Occasional snakes rustled beneath her yurt. As she made mental lists for the tasks of the next day—either minor repairs of the facilities, shopping, or fulfilling special requests for ritual instruments—sometimes her mind wandered to the sensation of what it would feel like if a rattler sank its teeth into her flesh. She imagined it would be something like being pierced by a fiery brand.

"I would try to catch them in the middle of the night," she said. Snakes are cold-blooded and much less likely to bite when the sun is down. She lashed metal roofing strips to her cowboy boots and arms to protect herself from the fangs and, thus armored, she fished under the small platform between the yurt and the ground with a crooked stick. It would bang against the mortar foundations but never managed to hook a snake. They stuck around. Either she would have to make her peace with them or bring in a professional to round them up.

With nothing to show for her efforts, Moore would stand up in her makeshift suit of armor and gaze into the sky and take in a calming breath. In the distance, she could make out the sounds of pickup trucks barreling down a distant highway and blasting country music. "I had a great time," she remembered.

Among her chores was the responsibility to deliver food to every retreatant's yurt. The encampment was about a mile away from where she put up. Like everyone under Roach's administration, she had endless rules to follow. She wasn't allowed to speak with any of the retreatants except through letters. She had to avoid eye contact or risk polluting their meditations with impressions of the outside world, so she hauled supplies to the five yurts as quietly as possible. On her very first visit she realized that one of the structures was empty. McNally was sharing a room with Roach. After the scene at her vow ceremony, the coupling didn't surprise her, but she also knew it wasn't part of the plan.

For the people under her care the days quickly fell into a rhythm that started with early-morning meditation and yoga and then a light breakfast. McNally and Roach ate out of the same bowl of Cheerios. In the afternoon they did another set of meditation practices, and then, as evening fell, McNally translated texts from the ACIP archive. Roach began working on his next book. The texts they drew from invoked violent and wrathful deities whose rage would help them cut through their ignorance and obstacles to enlightenment. They studied how harnessing their own sexual energies could enhance their meditative states. They hoped to take on the qualities of their divine protectors so that they would be able to see the people around them as angels. Having grown up in a different Buddhist tradition, Moore was skeptical about their process.

Almost a decade after the retreat ended, she said, "Most lamas don't have the amount of pride that it would actually take to read one of these books and think, 'Oh yes, I am totally qualified to start to do this without any additional instruction.' I mean, nobody would do that. Nobody that I know other than Geshe Michael would do that. Even if they could read all the books, they would never propose to think that they could actually do it without having had the transmission of specific permission or instruction."

Since it began in 1995, the ACIP had digitized tens of thousands of Tibetan texts so that the combined knowledge of thousands of masters was only a few keystrokes away. This meant that retreatants had access to one of the most extensive databases of esoteric spiritual knowledge in the world. Many of the books hadn't been looked at in hundreds of years.

In earlier generations, texts were hard to come by, and Buddhist practitioners paid dearly for whatever knowledge they could find that would connect them to the masters of the past. In medieval times, a monk might walk for years over the Himalayas to retrieve a single text to meditate on. The digital revolution that Roach helped usher in had changed the relationship between dharma practitioners and the rarified knowledge they sought. It was Enlightenment 2.0 and the spiritual potential was immense. Roach and McNally sensed that the database offered them an advantage that had never before existed in history. With the stroke of a finger, they could bring up precise ancient instructions for any question that might arise during their three-year retreat.

In ancient Tibet the spiritual masters who pioneered thousand-day retreats recorded more than a few notes on their practices. There were sequences of prostrations, guided meditations, and mantra recitations designed to enable specific types of realizations in the consciousness of meditators. Realizations in Tibetan Buddhism are not supposed to come at random but, rather, in a particular sequence of increasing depth and profoundness. Ideally, it works like a machine.

Eventually the routine breaks down and the divisions between the devoted student's inner life, and the practices fade away. The practitioner simply *is*. What starts as watching air flow in and out of their own body builds over years of practice into understanding subtle energies flowing through a central channel of winds and energy. Time and discipline help dismantle the social and hereditary conditioning. All that's left is pure essence.

One of the most significant experiences that Tibetan meditators lay claim to is "seeing emptiness directly." This was the stage of enlightenment Michael Roach claimed to have come across while making tea for his master in New Jersey. Training for it begins with focusing one's attention on a single point and feeling the spaciousness of the mind itself. The experience of that spaciousness grows over years and builds into a relativistic state where all things are inherently empty of any sort of essential quality. The concept is simple enough to grasp on an intellectual level. Indeed, philosophers have chewed on it for thousands of years. But the meditator's aim is not intellectual; it's experiential. The gap between *knowing* emptiness and *being* emptiness is a river most people will never cross. The three-year retreat in Arizona was a sort of conditioning apparatus. A laboratory for emptiness.

Tantric texts are often cryptic in their meanings, and, like the ultimate reality that retreatants seek, the books don't present the complete message. Among Tibetan Buddhists, when a student learns a new text or technique, it is not enough simply to read the words on a page; the method must also be learned from a teacher who has already had authentic realizations. Buddhists describe the phenomenon of transmission as a direct link between the guru and the disciple. The guru was himself a disciple of another teacher, and the line, supposedly, goes all the way back to the Buddha.

To safeguard the authenticity of the knowledge, every teaching gets transmitted in three separate ways. The first is with an initiation, called *wang*, which empowers the prospective student to accept teachings on a spiritual level in the same way that a baptism works in Christianity to cleanse the spirit. The second part of transmission is the oral transmission, called *lung*—the same word as the wind energy that flows through the subtle body. The final step is *tri*, or the practical knowledge of the teaching, including mantras and the daily practices that the student has to adhere to. The components function as a safeguard against the theological drift that might happen if someone decides to reinterpret the spiritual lessons for their own purposes. When I asked the Buddhist scholar and journalist Matteo Pistono if it was ever okay to take teachings from a text without an initiation, he told me the only exception would be if the initiate was already a fully enlightened being. "You could only do that if you actually were [the goddess] Vajrayogini. In which case it would be like looking at your birth certificate and saying, 'This is me.' Otherwise it's just crazy." In other words, the initiation sanctifies a direct connection to some original divine inspiration, rather than the potential madness of a human hallucination.

The ACIP database was an archive of mostly forgotten materials; many of the books in it had not been read since they were placed on a moldering shelf in Mongolia or St. Petersburg. The vast majority of tantric works in the ACIP archive are texts without transmission. While useful for academic research, for a student, this is like having a lock without a key. Opening it requires grace from a higher power.

Divine revelation is a sticky problem in every faith. God, or whatever divine truth that adherents access, rarely speaks in a unified voice. Yet great religions strive to create universal edicts. On the other hand, mystics feed on idiosyncratic revelations. In his book *Under the Banner of Heaven,* Jon Krakauer noted how the Mormon Church struggled with divine revelations since its inception, after the prophet Joseph Smith encouraged his followers to seek instructions directly from God. Within a few years the doctrine had backfired. "Who was to say that the truths He revealed to Joseph had greater validity than

contradictory truths He might reveal to somebody else? With everyone receiving revelations, the prophet stood to lose control of his followers," writes Krakauer. The revelation problem fostered more than
two hundred schisms in the Church of Latter-Day Saints. A similar
dynamic helped spark the Protestant Reformation from Catholicism
and the countless denominations of modern-day evangelism.

Oral transmission helps keep Buddhism unified. A lineage that
goes unbroken from teacher to student back to the words of the Buddha is thought to contain an essential kernel of unbroken truth. The
master can watch the student have a mystical experience and rein
him in if he moves too far afield.

On the Great Retreat, Roach had access to an archive of lost knowledge that no other Tibetan Buddhist could claim an authentic link to.
Ownership made him the de facto steward. He could either leave the
texts frozen as scholarly relics of lost knowledge, or he could try to reclaim the knowledge from the texts through his own meditation.

So what he did not understand, Roach did his best to surmise by
filtering it through his years of training. He based the retreatants'
schedules on broad strokes of old methods and relied heavily on their
own divine inspiration and meditations to fill in the gaps. An outsider
might have said they were making it up as they went along. Roach
thought differently. He believed he was guided by angels.

For Roach the retreat was a way to blend the spiritual world of his
meditations with the ordinary world he lived in. Every day he brought
a vision of the goddess Vajrayogini to his mind and meditated on a
union with her. Sometimes he tried to see himself as the goddess. At
other times he joined with the goddess in sexual union. The barrier
between his visions and the ordinary world broke down when he realized that Christie McNally was a goddess. And not just any goddess, but an earthly emanation of Vajrayogini herself.

This breakthrough moment meant that instead of having sex
with a goddess in his mind, he could have sex with a goddess in real
life. While he preferred to never call it sex, Moore didn't have any
other word for it.

Roach and McNally threw the intensity of their practice into their relationship. Every moment was a challenge to merge two minds into one. It was an opportunity to merge their bodies too. They spent hours building up their sexual energy in what presumably was a hot and sweaty exercise that didn't end in release.

While it is impossible to know the exact practices that Roach and McNally pursued in the privacy of their own yurt, a survey of the existing literature on the subject, along with interviews with tantric yogis, makes it possible to reconstruct at least the broad themes. According to tantric logic, the moment of conception between a man and a woman involves both the physical connection of the sperm and the egg and an energetic connection of two subtle bodies that occurs during the moment of orgasm. The energies are so powerful that they explode into the germ of human life.* If repurposed away from conception, the energy could instead work toward any number of other goals. When two people who are already adept at meditation and yoga move their energies together, instead of channeling that force through ejaculation—which corresponds to the root chakra that controls the sex organs—they can shift the internal winds to experience the moment of release through the crown chakra at the top of the head. During the encounter, practitioners also maintain visualizations of a sort of final goal. That goal might be gaining wealth, finding love, a creative project, or anything else. As the energy streaks out of their crown chakras, it imbues their mental projection with the same generative forces that give birth to a new human life. If the practice was successful, it would plant a karmic seed for wishes to come true.

Roach and McNally's ordinary meditation practice involved intensive visualizations of various deities, but most important the goddess Vajrayogini. They would likely have been visualizing her above their heads while they projected their cosmic creative ejaculate into her form. Their goal was much more lofty than just growing rich, though. They wanted the goddess to give them transcendence. It was a sweaty spiritual mess. And, from the outside, about as hot as watch-

---

*Modern fertility techniques such as in vitro fertilization and egg donation, which have taken the moment of conception out of the bedroom and into the laboratory, would appear to complicate the energetic theory of human conception. However, the mysteries of the energetic world may be too subtle for us to ever understand rationally.

ing a balding fifty-ish man hold back his climax with a twentysomething woman.

· To enhance the experience, Roach adopted the symbols the goddess wears in *tangka* paintings to make them part of his real-world
identity. To embrace the goddess's feminine energy, Roach started
dressing in women's clothes. He stopped cutting his hair and let it
grow long, and wore bangles and a diamond stud earring that accen-
tuated his femininity.

Slowly, more people began to hear about strange things going on
inside the boundaries of the retreat. While Moore was the only person
living on the land full-time, other people interested in serving their
lama pitched in to do minor repairs, help with the cooking, and live
near the land. Though they were never likely to actually see the retreatants, they came from around the world to serve and accrue karmic
merit in their presence. If, in the course of their duties, they learned
something about their lama that didn't fit with their image of a whole-
some retreat, most had the good sense not to spread any rumors. Later,
one person who was considering ordination under Roach wrote an
anonymous blog entry and posted it online. "If, perhaps, I slipped into
a vision that this was in any way unethical for a monk, and certainly
more appealing for a 28 year old man, I quickly marked it down in my
little vow book as an infraction of my pure view." The unnamed writer
exposed how schisms began to form between the retreatants.

Rifts also formed inside the retreat itself. Susan Howler had long
black hair and sleepy eyes; everyone knew she had total devotion to
her lama. So it was a shock when she walked out of the retreat and
didn't look back. She had been inside for a year and a half, and an official account states that she had been sent away from the retreat on a
special mission. She was tight-lipped about what exactly happened,
but people close to her remember that she felt betrayed by Roach, and
her anger was directed specifically toward her teacher. In 2006, a
blogger on the website geshewatch, one of several websites maintained by Roach's ex-students, recounted that Howler and another
lady on the retreat told the writer that "Geshe Michael Roach, an ordained monk, had engaged in sexual activity with at least four of his

female students both before and during the retreat. Both claim that this sexual activity was mundane, rather than any form of holy consort practice, and included watching pornography, fellatio and more than one lady at the same time."*

If substantiated, the allegations threatened to put Roach in direct confrontation with the Geluk hierarchy. What would his teachers think about a veritable orgy happening under his watch? Roach had an inkling that he was treading on very dangerous ground and wanted to shore up support from the Tibetan community. Shortly before Christmas in 2003, he sent a letter to the office of the Dalai Lama in India as well as to other influential Tibetan teachers. He also posted it online. In retrospect, it was so blind to the political realities of the moment that there is no doubt it was written in complete earnestness.

In the letter, Roach asked the Dalai Lama to write a blurb for the book he had been working on in his yurt. He also came clean about the irregularities in his practice, hoping that the leader in the Tibetan order would embrace his unorthodox actions. Roach declared that he had grasped the nature of emptiness directly and that Christie McNally had helped him get there. He called her the Diamond Queen, admitted he had begun to dress as the goddess, and asked for recognition of the feat.

The Dalai Lama refused to respond, nor would he offer any of his words to be used as promotional material for Roach's books. Instead, the letter circulated online and in the listings of official communications of the Dalai Lama. However, Lama Zopa Rinpoche, the founder

---

*I contacted Howler in 2012 and 2013 and she categorically denied that the blog posts and testimony from multiple sources are anything more than rumor. She wrote to me the following statement:

> Geshe Michael and Christie lived together in their own private yurt, and each of us had our own separate yurts. We only met occasionally during that time, usually like every other month for a handful of times, and always as a group. These women are all very close friends of mine, for over 15 years now, and I never heard any of them talk about or even hint of anything strange going on.
>
> Of these women, two are nuns who continue to teach and do retreats in the Buddhist lineage, and two (including myself) are laypeople who maintain a positive relationship with Geshe Michael and continue to be involved in teaching and spreading Buddhist teachings. To the best of my knowledge, none of us have ever made any statement that we had any type of sexual or intimate relationship with Geshe Michael, or that we have been hurt by him as a teacher in any way.

of the FPMT, did comment. In an open letter, he asked whether Roach was confused about what he had learned on retreat. Maybe the monk in Arizona had succumbed to his delusions rather than achieving advanced states of consciousness. To tell the difference, he suggested a simple test. Roach could prove himself by demonstrating his powers in front of a wide audience, and, given the sexual overtones, preferably with his penis. To preserve modesty, Zopa substituted the Tibetan word for thunderbolt, *vajra*, for the English word *cock*.

If one performs those behaviors to develop people's devotion then it is not just an ordinary miracle that is needed. One needs to do a special kind of miracle. For example the 6th Dalai Lama pee-ed from the top of the Potala and just before the urine hit the ground he drew it back again inside his vajra. Also there is the story of the previous incarnation of Gonsar Rinpoche who pulled in mud through his vajra. This is just my suggestion I don't know what other Lamas and Gurus will advise.

With much love and prayers, Lama Zopa

Whether Roach was still following the ancient wisdoms or simply improvising his own spiritual path is academic, but the transformation would have an impact on his following. Approximately every six months from the time they entered the retreat, Roach and the other retreatants emerged from the silence to give public talks about their experiences.

In the absence of Roach himself, many of the day-to-day decisions at Diamond Mountain were made by a specially appointed board of directors. These administrators and donors were people who were loyal to Roach and accepted the potential liability that came with having their names listed on the state paperwork for the organization. In some ways, it's no surprise that Diamond Mountain was organized like a corporation.

His first mass-market book, *The Diamond Cutter: The Buddha on Managing Your Business and Your Life*, had become a bestseller in the first months of the Great Retreat. Thousands of people around the world were eager to start studying with the monk who had made a fortune in the diamond business. To protect the retreatants from outside influences, the board of directors, who oversaw the administrative functions of Diamond Mountain, held the Great Retreat teachings in a room that was divided down the middle by a large curtain. The retreatants sat on one side, the lay community on the other. Susan Howler refused to attend the teachings, and the board members made excuses that she was away on urgent spiritual business. When it was their turn to lecture, the retreatants wore blindfolds on stage so they would not have to have their minds polluted by the outside world. Thousands tuned in to the live webstream, and thousands more downloaded the recordings. To certify the achievement of three years in silence, Roach bequeathed the title "lama" on all of the women who emerged from the retreat. McNally was the only one to affix the title to her name officially.

On the last teaching of the last day of the talks, Lama Christie McNally climbed onto the stage like the angel that Roach had declared her to be. She wore all-white robes with a scarf draped over her neck and seemed to float lightly on her pedestal. A golden silk blindfold covered her eyes. She began her talk with a short meditation and there was an electric energy flowing through the audience as they anticipated her revelations.

Before she entered the retreat, she said, she wanted to find enlightenment. She wanted to save the world. The retreat had let her grow in profound ways and there were long moments when she achieved that elusive goal of single-pointed concentration. The emptiness was almost palpable, angels everywhere. Despite all this, the most important thing she learned was something that she knew going in: Her lama had power. She began to tell a story—a hypothetical one, she said—but it sounded suspiciously like a peek into her private relationship with Roach.

Imagine, she said, that they were sitting by a fire beneath the stars with desert crickets chirping in the distance. In this idyllic setting, Roach asked her to test her faith. "If I had a student they could put their hand right in that fire," he said. Christie trusted Roach, but the fire scared her. Logic told her that it would singe her skin. The flesh would peel back in layers of pain. She played out her mental conversation.

Why would this be a good thing to do? To follow my lama's advice and stick my hand into this fire? Well, he is a perfectly infallible being who has so much love for me that I can't even understand it. All he wants is to get me enlightened in this life. All he wants is for me to see emptiness directly.

And so you get the faith you need, and you stick your hand into the fire. And what happens, funny thing, your hand, it doesn't burn. It doesn't burn. You're sitting there with your hand in the fire, and flames are all around you, and it doesn't burn. So it's an object lesson on emptiness, right? It's the emptiness of fire's ability to burn you. It's the emptiness of your hand's ability to feel the fire. It's the emptiness of your awareness of the two of those coming together. But it's also a miracle, you know, brought about by your faith. That's all. Thank you.

—Lama Christie McNally, April 20, 2003

As she got up from the stage and walked blindfolded back into the partitioned side of the tent the audience gasped at the recitation of the miracle. Had the retreat been a success? Had Roach mastered what he had come to do? Had McNally?

To find out, a Buddhist monk named T. Monkyi from outside the Diamond Mountain community traveled to the retreat teachings to interview Roach and McNally. He had read the letters and believed he would be able to publish the interview in a Buddhist magazine. As far as I've been able to tell, the article was never published. However, a twenty-five-page transcript of the interview has circulated online since then. It offers the most transparent account that Roach and McNally gave after they finished the Great Retreat. It was probably the last unfiltered interview Roach ever offered the press.

Little is known about T. Monkyi's identity, but the transcript shows him to be at least as well versed in Tibetan Buddhist theology as Roach. He was skeptical of the claims the two made and questioned them on their break with tradition.

Roach explained that it was too easy to get caught up in salacious details of tantric sex and miss the more important point. After all, that aspect of their relations was a lot "like doing yoga for four hours a day or five hours a day; it's not fun. And it's not a joke. It's a life-or-death attempt to become a being who can serve all living creatures before you die."

Roach implored Monkyi to understand that he had prayed for Vajrayogini to appear to him for his whole life. He wanted to see her with his own eyes. To touch her. When he first experienced a taste of emptiness in his twenties, he set his intention to meet the goddess. Now that he had her in his arms, he wasn't about to let her go, no matter what a distant Buddhist hierarchy half a world away might think.

Roach continued:

I honestly believe that it is more important for me to do what a divine being might indicate for me is important for me to do than [worry about] all of the impressions that people might have. . . . If a lot of people thought I was being a bad person, or a bad monk, or even a corrupt person, that was less important than doing what I felt a divine being wanted me to do, even if everyone thought it was crazy. I've never had a doubt about that. I think that it's more important for me to get enlightened and to follow what I perceive to be direct divine instructions than to be thought of as a bad person.

The Great Retreat broke the hierarchy between Roach and Tibetan authorities. Now that he was under the direct guidance of angels, there was no need to appeal to the Dalai Lama. With Lama Christie by his side, he promised they would breathe new life into Tibetan Buddhism. They would forge a faith that shucked off anachronistic Tibetan traditions and make their interpretation of ancient Buddhist wisdom relevant for modern-day America.

Part 2

Sacred Spaces

The Buddha and the Ferryboat

THE HEADWATERS OF the holy Ganga River start in the high Himalayas where snow collects in the crevices of the ancient range. When the year turns hot, the snows melt, and great torrents of water rush down across the plains in a journey that inevitably leads to the sea. When the mountains are in their wettest mood, travelers find it difficult to cross the web of tributaries and streams that wash across the land. In the eras before industrialization, the situation made the job of ferryman potentially lucrative. With a few sturdy pieces of wood and a stout rope that spanned the width of one particularly troublesome stream, a man could eke out a living bringing travelers from one side of the water to another. Depending on how wild the water was, or how old and withered the rope puller on the boat might be, a trip could take a long time. So it was not uncommon to have many people waiting on either side of a crossing for their turn on the raft.

One day the Buddha was walking along one such swollen tributary and he came upon a crowded crossing. The ferryman had already departed the Buddha's bank and was on his way to the other side. The Buddha sat down and waited. A moment passed and then the Buddha noticed a wiry old ascetic with long matted hair sitting nearby. The Rishi was covered in ash and had long strands of holy beads around his neck. He wore a loincloth around his waist, and his eyes burned with intensity.

When their eyes met, the Rishi proclaimed that he was a devotee of the great lord Shiva and had spent a quarter century practicing austerities in his honor. The Rishi said he slept exposed to the elements and covered himself in the ashes collected from funeral pyres. Every day he deprived himself of the bounty of life so that he could seek a divine reward from his lord. The Buddha was intrigued and asked what the Rishi had received so far.

The Rishi cast a proud smile at the Buddha. "Behold!" he said. The Rishi sprang to his feet and sprinted toward the swollen river. He launched himself over the water, but instead of plunging below the current, his feet touched the liquid as if he was on solid land. The old man walked across the river and his feet did not even make a splash. When he was on the other side he looked back at the Buddha and chortled. The Buddha could offer no such trick.

The Buddha sat on his riverbank with his eyes as steady as a lake on a summer morning. In time the ferryman returned. The Buddha handed the puller a penny and let the old man take him to the opposite side. The Rishi was still grinning, sure that the Buddha would bow to him and recognize Shiva as the most powerful deity of all. But the Buddha returned the Rishi's gaze with pity.

"So much wasted time!" the Buddha lamented. "After twenty-five years of devotion, you received the power to walk on water, but to what end? All I needed to cross was a penny."

9.

Sacred Spaces

Wisdom sits in places. It's like water that never dries up. You need to drink water to stay alive, don't you? Well, you also need to drink from places. You must remember everything about them. You must learn their names. You must remember what happened at them long ago. You must think about it and keep on thinking about it. Then your mind will become smoother and smoother. Then you will see danger before it happens.
— Dudley Patterson, a Chiricahua Apache horseman

The worst place of all is Apache Pass. There, five Indians, one my brother, were murdered. Their bodies were hung up and kept there till they were skeletons.
— Cochise, chief of the Chiricahua Apache

THE MORMON RANCHER who owned the land where Roach and Mc-Nally first established Diamond Mountain University was eager to reclaim the plot for his own use. Once they completed their thousand-day retreat in the desert, he gently suggested the Buddhists find another place to stay. So, for a time, the couple wandered the globe, lecturing on the nature of love and karma, and relied on the charity of their students for room and board. But transience did not suit them.

They yearned not only to regain what they had lost but to establish a permanent base. Together they dreamed of making Diamond Mountain more than a university in name only. They wanted a campus with a tantric college, retreat cabins, and study centers dedicated to promoting Roach's lineage. The buildings would be energy efficient and designed to blend into the landscape; there would be solar panels and rainwater harvesting. It could be paradise on earth. The university would last a thousand years.

The search for a new space took five years. Then, in 2008, the board members of Diamond Mountain finalized the paperwork on the deed for a parcel of land about eighty miles east of St. David. The plot stood directly adjacent to Fort Bowie, a decaying garrison that was once the center for military operations against the Apache. The previous owner called the property Bear Creek Ranch, and it had some obvious advantages over the first location: For one, the lot actually had a mountain within its borders. The hulking walls of rock offered privacy that the open range had not. When they arrived, a spring of fresh water flowed strong enough to feed a herd of cattle.

The 960-acre plot cost $1.1 million, which Roach raised through speaking fees and donations from the wealthier members of his flock. Christie McNally was delighted that the board would actually own land instead of renting it. The money was a down payment on the future spiritual progress of Buddhism in America.

A small hill between imposing mountains divided the valley into two campuses. The entrance would house the basic-support administrative buildings that would become the public face of the university. They began building a temple, a house for Roach to live in, and several yurts and kitchen facilities. Guests could set up tents on the other side of a dry wash that ran parallel to the main access road. They filled the gravel parking lot with temporary trailers, which stank of stale coffee and sewage, for support staff to live in. With money, time, and hard work, everything would get upgraded.

The interior valley would be altogether different. There, Roach's followers began to construct retreat cabins that were isolated from the rest of the world. The structures were specifically designed for meditation and meant to blend into and enhance the landscape as much as possible.

On the far side of the retreat valley a vertical slope of loose gravel and cacti ascends more than one thousand feet. Caves left by prospectors and clefts in the rock marked the mountain's face. They dubbed the mountain Tara Mountain after a Tibetan goddess. At its summit the new owners hung a string of green, yellow, red, and white prayer flags inscribed with Tibetan script. Tibetans believe that as the wind blows over the flags' sacred lettering, prayers of peace and enlightenment float over the valley. From the summit, a person could also see the flagpole at Fort Bowie, a powerful reminder that settling here wasn't just a legal or financial affair. Before the Buddhists arrived to found the second incarnation of their university, and for as long as anyone could remember, this land had always been bought with violence. In a way, the forces that drive conflict might be as old as the land itself.

Twenty-seven million years ago a small cone of congealed magma built up on a weak point in the earth's crust and stuck in the ground like a cork just two miles south of the valley that Diamond Mountain now occupies. Countless centuries of continental movements and subterranean lava flows pushed upward against the plug until the pressure was released in an explosion of volcanic ash and magma a thousand times more powerful than the eruption at Mount St. Helens. The hot cloud darkened the globe and robbed plants in faraway Indonesia and Germany of sunlight and caused chaos in global weather patterns for decades. For Southeast Arizona, this might as well have been the moment of creation.

The cataclysm erased any trace of what came before it. The mountain's once-mighty peak collapsed in an instant into a twelve-mile-wide volcanic crater that now descends almost a mile into the earth at its deepest point. Ash that settled outside of ground zero left behind a Mars-like landscape. Over the following eons ice, wind, and excoriating sun sculpted the softer minerals away and left behind improbable rock shapes. Spires of hardened magma that resemble carefully stacked pebbles, called hoodoos, can soar hundreds of feet into the air. At the heart of the caldera, their trunklike pinnacles form a forest of rock pillars.

The native people who first settled near the shell of the volcano discovered a natural fortress. Mineral-rich flatlands on either side of the range helped grow crops of beans and maize. In times of danger, prehistoric inhabitants retreated to cliffside dwellings and staged carefully planned ambushes on invaders who didn't have an intimate knowledge of the terrain. For the people at Diamond Mountain the natural privacy ensured by the rock formations was an asset as they pursued higher realizations. The valley's steep walls made it difficult for all but the most determined visitors to peek in on their affairs.

The only two springs that bubble to the surface in the Chiricahua Mountains are just north of the extinguished volcano. They sit less than half a mile from each other. One, called Apache Spring, is on land owned and operated by the National Park Service under Fort Bowie. The other, called Bear Spring, struggles to the surface in the heart of the retreat valley.

The presence of water allowed life to flourish here in a way that it never could in the rest of the range. It also made the land holy in the eyes of the Apache, who were normally nomadic and lived in hastily thatched-together domes, called wickiups, that could be constructed quickly and torn down without a trace. Access to fresh water tempered the Apache's wanderlust. As one of the few places the Apache chose to continuously inhabit, the springs were some of the most sacred locations in their cosmology.

The most prominent and violent of the five or six major Apache tribes were the Chiricahua. Apache Spring was at the heart of their ancestral range. Led by fearsome warriors who believed they were the recipients of a divine blessing known as *power*, the Chiricahua gained a reputation for perseverance against long odds and a willingness to protect what was theirs. The anthropologist M. E. Opler, who spent much of his life studying the Apache, wrote that power was "a mighty force that pervades the universe. Some of it filters through to the hands of man."

For some Apache, power was an avenue to cure disease, or to locate water. For others it gave them strength in battle. Warriors imbued with it could raise dust storms to confound their enemies and hide the trail of their war party or confer immunity to weapons. While all Apache shared the belief in power, for the Chiricahua, it was their lifeblood. David Roberts, a biographer of several prominent Apache warriors, wrote, "Because of the ubiquity of these supernatural gifts among the people, Indians from other tribes concluded that all the Chiricahua were witches."

Though they come from different roots, Apache spirituality and Tibetan Buddhism have certain synergies that Roach and McNally frequently mentioned. Both the Apache and Roach believed it was possible to cultivate supernatural abilities, and both groups had a sense of sacred geography. Tibetans believe that sages from the past could hide secret spiritual teachings, called treasures, in geographic features—writing the words of the Buddha in the face of the mountain or in the clouds for later prophets to discover during their meditations. Anthropologist Keith Basso once wrote that the Apache say "wisdom sits in places," by which he meant that the Chiricahua believe that land remembers its own history, and a careful observer can learn lessons about future dangers by watching the landscape.

If the land beneath Diamond Mountain remembers only one date, it would be February 5, 1861, when Lieutenant George Bascom, a brash Union officer who graduated twenty-sixth out of twenty-seven in his class at West Point, made camp near Apache Spring. In the preceding century, American settlers practiced a brutal campaign of extermination and pacification against native peoples. This part of Arizona had only recently become a U.S. territory, and Bascom wanted the Indians on this land to understand what it meant to be under American rule. Officially, however, Bascom came to Apache Spring to speak to the Chiricahua chief Cochise about the disappearance of a young boy named Felix Ward.

Twice Bascom's age of twenty-five, Cochise had taut muscles and carried himself with the dignity of a statesman. Three brass rings hung from his ears and he was so constantly serious that even his closest friends had never seen him smile. In a gesture of good faith, Cochise arrived at Bascom's camp with his brother, wife, two children, and two nephews in tow. The Kentuckian offered them coffee.

As the chief and soldier exchanged pleasantries, Bascom's men quietly surrounded the tent and leveled their rifles at its entrance.

Sure that he had the upper hand, Bascom accused Cochise of kidnapping Ward and demanded that Cochise return the child or face the full might of the U.S. Army. Cochise remained calm, explaining that he had no knowledge of the raid on the nearby ranch—indeed, this was the truth; Ward surfaced a decade later to report that he had been taken prisoner by another tribe. Cochise promised that he would help the lieutenant find the missing child, but the profession of innocence was not enough. The officer said he would hold Cochise and his family hostage until the child was returned. If Cochise resisted, then his soldiers were ready to fire.

Cochise didn't stop to weigh his options. His hand came down onto the hilt of his knife and he sprang to his feet. In one swift motion, he cut a long slash in the canvas tent and before Bascom could draw his revolver, he bolted through the gaping hole. He sprinted across the valley floor, dodging and weaving through scrub brush. The soldiers fired fifty shots from pistols and rifles. When the smoke from their gunpowder cleared, they saw Cochise bounding straight up the mountainside, limping only slightly because a bullet had grazed his leg. It all happened so fast that when Cochise looked down, he saw that the coffee cup was still in his hand.

The Chiricahua remember Cochise's escape by the name cut-the-tent. Settlers called it the Bascom Affair. The betrayal set off a series of bloody reprisals between the Apache and Arizona ranchers that would claim more than a thousand lives. Bascom hung Cochise's brother from a tree at Apache Pass. It was left there as a warning to any Apache who resisted. Birds picked at his body until it slowly decayed and fell apart.

In return, Cochise vowed that he would slaughter every rancher he came across and used the rocky natural defenses to murderous advantage. Cochise started raiding ranches and wagon trains in the new territory, often torturing his victims to death. A year after hostilities broke out, he learned that a large contingent of soldiers was going to leave the garrison in Tucson to reinforce Union troops in the Civil War that was being waged in the East. Since it was the only source of water for many days' ride, Cochise knew that the soldiers would have to resupply themselves at Apache Spring.

Cochise brought together the largest force of Apache warriors ever assembled to meet them. Five hundred Apache hid behind rocks and in natural caves on the mountainside, all along Apache Pass and back into the valley that now belongs to Diamond Mountain. The Indians marked the soldiers' slow progress by the dust that their horses and wagons kicked up. The cloud grew in the sky until the parched soldiers came into sight, but Cochise urged his troops to hold their fire.

They waited until the approaching troop was just six hundred yards short of the spring before they opened fire. The initial salvo dropped two men in blue uniforms and the battle continued for three hours, with both sides shooting from behind cover. Cochise had the high ground and the element of surprise, but he didn't know what to make of the strange-looking wagons the soldiers dragged to the front lines. The Apache had never seen cannon before, and when the twelve-pound howitzers bombarded their positions, at least nine Apache died. What should have been an easy victory turned into a rout. "After they turned cannon loose on us at Apache Pass, my people were certain that they were doomed," he said later. The Indians fled without the taste of victory.

Wary of ever having to face a similar attack by Indians again, the army erected Fort Bowie at Apache Pass in 1862. The low adobe structures overlooked the spring to the south and soon became the headquarters for all anti-Indian operations in that part of Arizona. Cochise fled across the open plain to a bulwark of impenetrable rock formations in a place now called Cochise Stronghold almost fifty miles away. From there he was limited to small raids and never gathered a force large enough to mount another head-on attack on the army.

The resistance continued unabated for decades in increasing spates of tit-for-tat violence. Settlers murdered Apache holy men in cold blood, and thousands of renegade Apache were rounded up as prisoners and slaughtered. The few who fled the small reservations that sprang up from time to time continued their guerrilla fight. Eventually, Cochise died and an Apache recluse named Geronimo replaced him, if not as chief of the tribe, then as its most prized warrior.

Geronimo was short, with dark, brutal features. He wore his hair long, and his wide nose gave him a grim demeanor. At about 170 pounds, he was stocky and powerfully built. In the most famous photograph ever taken of an Indian, a picture that hangs in the cloakroom of the temple at Diamond Mountain, Geronimo kneels down, holding a short rifle, with his eyes burning with the wrath of a man who saw his tribe all but vanquished. Where Cochise was regal and patient, Geronimo was quick to anger and often drunk and unreasonable. Early in his life he went on a vision quest in the mountains above Fort Bowie, where he took peyote and earned a power that the Apache called enemy against. The great spirit Ussen came to him and prophesied that Geronimo would never fall in battle, but also that he would not die on Apache land. Years later, his son Juh, a great warrior in his own right, remembered Geronimo's power this way (as quoted by David Roberts):

> He was by nature already a brave person; but if one knows he will never be killed in battle, why be afraid? I don't know that Geronimo ever told his warriors that he had supernatural protection, but they were with him in many dangerous times and saw his miraculous escapes, his cures for wounds and the results of his medicine; so his warriors knew that Geronimo was only alive because of Ussen's protection.

Geronimo's resistance movement was smaller, but also more deadly, than Cochise's. He brought together a handful of fighters—all women and men who were said to have power of their own. For twenty-eight years they roamed from Northern Mexico to Northern Arizona on the warpath, occasionally circling back to an Indian reservation established at Apache Pass. Every week his band struck a new ranch, wagon train, or lone rancher. They'd plunder the ammunition and supplies from the victims, rape the women, and murder the men. Sometimes he tortured them, sometimes he didn't. He would throw babies into the air and skewer them on his bayonet. It was revenge for the ill treatment of the Indians. As he grew older and more experienced, his warriors saw his powers mature. He seemed to have the ability to divine events that were happening many miles away. They said he could intuit the enemies' movements before they did.

As the numbers of dead continued to climb, capturing Geronimo became a top priority for the U.S. government. Once the Civil War was over, they deployed a quarter of what remained of the army to the Arizona Territory. More than five thousand soldiers flooded the state. Soldiers seemed to be everywhere, but Geronimo evaded them with ease. The soldiers installed a revolutionary new heliograph system—a precursor to the telegraph—to track Geronimo's movements and kill him. Yet Geronimo and his band of just twelve warriors proved to be more than a match for the legions that chased him. His bloody campaign continued until 1886—a stretch of outlawry that seems almost impossible today. Low estimates say that Geronimo personally killed twenty-five people, but some claim that he and his band took the lives of more than five hundred. When he had reached the age of fifty-seven, he had fought against the whites for his whole life. He was tired. He surrendered in Mexico to a small group of soldiers who had come to negotiate peace, and on April 2 of that year he was brought back to Fort Bowie and held prisoner before being sent to live out his days on a reservation far away from his homeland.

Stories of Geronimo and Cochise were never far from the lips of people at Diamond Mountain. At times it felt to them as if the new university was following in Indian footsteps and bringing spiritual existence back to the land of the vanquished Indians. In 2007, even before the final cash payment was settled for the plot, the board of Diamond Mountain announced that they would attempt to make amends for the crimes of their ancestors through a special ceremony.

On their official blog, they wrote, "For many generations the land we now call Diamond Mountain was home to the Apache people. When outside forces came to remove these people there was a struggle and bloodshed. Many terrible things happened on the land and Diamond Mountain wants to make things right and purify those actions." They brought an Apache shaman to oversee the ceremony and implore the Apache spirits to pass custodianship of the land to the university.

More than a hundred years later, it is hard to see how the bloodshed was worth it. Cochise County is only sparsely populated, with little to show of industrial development, educational achievement, or economic output. Just fifty miles of uninhabited wasteland and dry mountain ridgelines from the Mexican border, the valley lies in a well-known drug smuggling corridor. The smugglers carry their contraband in backpacks and travel mostly by night, and their abandoned campsites decay in shallow washes and mountain caves. When border patrol agents and National Park rangers come across the narcoleros, there are often fierce confrontations, occasionally leaving one party or the other injured or dead. For the most part, though, the smugglers prefer to stay under the radar and out of sight. The United States would not have lost much had it left the land in the hands of the Apache.

Instead, Cochise County became a home for fringe religious groups that want to be left on their own and don't mind living in the desolate environment in exchange for privacy. Mormons who fled to St. David found solace in its emptiness. Others saw the privacy as a right and, like the Apache, took up arms to defend their imperiled beliefs. A few notable clashes between law enforcement and radical religious groups have left the local sheriff's department hesitant to meddle with anything that happens under the auspices of religion.

South of Sierra Vista, only a short drive from Fort Bowie on a lonesome stretch of Arizona State Route 92, a fire-and-brimstone preacher named Asa Alonzo Allen bought twenty-five hundred acres of desert land in 1958 and dubbed it Miracle Valley. Thousands would come to hear his sermons, witness his healing powers, and bask in the grace of a Christian god. The compound spawned the headquarters of an evangelical radio station, a summer camp, and a Bible college. Its congregation raised annual revenues of more than $2.5

million. When Allen died of complications related to alcoholism in San Francisco in 1970, the campus languished until 1978. In that year a black preacher, Reverend Frances Thomas from Chicago, took over much of the property. The church brought a sense of persecution with it to Arizona. Wary of Arizona's racist reputation, the church armed its members and sent out security teams with shotguns to patrol the property.

The Cochise County sheriff stepped in to mediate the brewing dispute but only seemed to exacerbate the situation. Among the church's teachings was the belief that God was responsible for both healing and sickness, and when church members became sick, they relied on faith instead of medicine. (Roach also teaches that all sickness has a divine origin and an equally divine cure.) In 1981, four children in the community got sick and died. The county believed that the deaths could have been prevented if the congregation had given them medicine. When the county attempted to remove other children from the compound and place them under state care, the already unstable situation turned violent.

One morning, the police arrested two members of the church's congregation for being unruly, but Thomas's flock thought the charges were unjust so they donned their Sunday best and loaded into a van that resembled the one driven by the A-Team. They were carrying bombs made of dynamite and cheap timers with plans to blow a hole in the jail's wall. As they drove down the county road, one of the timers shorted and the dynamite exploded. One man died, and the other two passengers were injured and sprayed with bits of flesh from his body. "The worst part of the explosion was having to swallow two mouthfuls of Brother Stevie," said one female occupant.

There were arrests, but the sheriff's department couldn't stem the resentment between the black church and the mostly white community. Then in October 1982, three dozen cops descended on the compound with the intention of serving traffic warrants to some of the church members. Thomas suspected a raid and her people armed themselves with bats, clubs, and rifles. A local AP photographer captured the ensuing fight. Black church members confronted the po-

lice, and the scared cops opened fire. The standoff ended when two
church members were killed, including Thomas's son. Five deputies
were hurt and one later died. Photographs from the shoot-out ended
up on the front page of *The New York Times*. Jesse Jackson and Reverend Al Sharpton came to Cochise County and charged the police
with aggravating an already dangerous situation.

The shoot-out is the most famous black mark on the Cochise
County Sheriff's Department's permanent record. Some cops there
still have the jobs they had thirty years ago and still speak fondly of
their fallen comrades. They remember the confrontation and are reluctant to interfere with any religious groups that set up shop. No
matter how strange things got at the churches nearby, the county
would rather leave them alone than risk another shoot-out. When the
odd group of Tibetan Buddhists showed up outside Fort Bowie, the
sheriff chose not to repeat earlier mistakes and gave Diamond Mountain a wide berth.

In 2007, Roach and McNally climbed up a hill that overlooked
what would become Diamond Mountain property, with an Apache
holy man. The moment they saw the valley, they knew it was perfect,
but were wary of offending the spiritual legacy of the place. In years
past, soldiers used the hill to track the movements of Indians. Fallen
rifle cartridges still poked out of the crags and up from the sandy soil
here. The small group sat together and lit a sacred fire. They burned
sage and aromatic herbs and sang songs to the Apache god Ussen for
permission to use the valley. The ceremony would help heal the land.
Some people remember that the shaman threw cash into the fire: fifteen thousand dollars to pay back centuries of violence. Chants
echoed off the valley walls throughout the day and into the night.
When they were exhausted and all that was left were the embers of
the ceremony's sacred fire, the troupe climbed back down the mountain in the hope that Ussen had accepted their gift.

A quarter mile away in the heart of what would be the retreat
valley, Bear Spring had bubbled forth from the earth for centuries.
For as long as any rancher, soldier, or Apache warrior could remember, it was a source of life in the hostile desert and fed from the same

subterranean flows that kept Apache Spring alive. As Diamond Mountain laid foundations for their university and hastened construction of the retreat center, silt began to fill in the water source. The flow withered to a trickle. Within a year the spring had dried up. Some people said it was a sign.

10.

Twelve Years, Fifteen Feet

I did not marry Geshe Michael because I was in love with him. And he did not marry me because he was in love with me. That was not the nature of our relationship. He was my lama. And for him I was an emanation of a divine being.

—Christie McNally

THERE IS NO WAY to know for sure how many vows Christie Mc-Nally and Michael Roach exchanged on their wedding day. Habituated to accepting monk and layperson commitments, tantric vows, and monastic mandates by the hundreds, the couple believed that the more rules they followed, the more perfect they would become. One vow was inescapably public and not found anywhere in Buddhist literature: From their marriage onward, the monk and his wife promised to never be more than fifteen feet apart from each other. McNally followed in Roach's footsteps wherever he went. On airplanes, when one would go to the bathroom, the other would have to wait outside the door so they would not break their spiritual bond. Every private meeting, dark night of the soul, and public speech was a test of their commitment. They hoped to forge a single being out of two people. It was a perfect love that defied the rational limits of human relationships. Both Roach and McNally believed in the possibility of perfection, and the crucible of constant contact inspired audiences around the world.

From an objective standpoint, it was a success. When they were side by side, attendance at events and lectures was never higher. They taught together, and their mutual confidence and earnestness seemed like an open door to the divine realm. The message was that enlightenment didn't have to be an isolating mission; you could take a spiritual partner along for the ride. Couples joined and worked on meditating together. Sex was a spiritual practice.

Roach and McNally became members of the jet set almost immediately after they left the first Great Retreat. Patrons flew them from Arizona to New York, and everywhere they went—from Germany and Russia to Singapore and Mexico—massive crowds turned out to meet them. McNally dressed in long, white flowing robes, and they gave teachings together on elevated thrones in rented churches, in corporate boardrooms, and at Asian Classics Institute properties around the world. They offered relationship advice based on the law of karma. They cowrote books and cultivated ties with wealthy donors who sought any spiritual validation that outrageous profits were a sign of good karma.

When in Manhattan, the small Three Jewels bookstore didn't fit the image they were trying to project anymore. No longer aiming at the hippie crowd that delighted in shabby-chic coffee tables and cast-off furniture, they instead booked lecture spaces in upscale spas and tasteful yoga studios that marketed to stressed-out Wall Street power brokers. On one trip east, they took a cab up to Columbia University, where the Tibetan scholar Robert Thurman held court. As an officiant at the first Tibetan Freedom Concert, the best-known translator of *The Tibetan Book of the Dead,* and a close friend of the Dalai Lama, Thurman had the power to lend credibility to Roach's spiritual path.

Years later Thurman was still angry about the encounter. He had come to believe that Roach's infractions weren't only a slight to his own training and credentials but were a serious threat to the larger Tibetan Buddhist community. His voice barked into ever higher registers as he recounted their meeting over the phone. "I told him that you can't be a monk and have a girlfriend. You have clearly given up your vow. To which he responded that he had never had genital contact with a human being. So I turned to her and asked her if she was human or not. And then there was a pregnant pause, and then she said, 'I can be whatever he wants me to be because he has realized emptiness.'" The scholar considered his words and sighed. Then he added, "They had already declined into psychosis."

The audiences didn't seem to care that Roach wasn't holding the Geluk line. To them Roach was either a reformer breaking anachronistic traditions or, for people who had never studied Tibetan Buddhism, a conduit directly back to the knowledge spoken by the Buddha. Mercedes Bahleda had been one of Roach's and McNally's closest attendants since the days when the Asian Classics Institute was nothing more than a series of free lectures in Manhattan parks. She saw Roach's insurrection as a feminist enterprise. "[Roach] couldn't give his young female students what they needed, so he made a conscious decision to fill that void by pouring his lineage into Christie and creating a female lama for the world," she said. It was true that women in particular had a difficult time finding a place in the Tibetan hierarchy. Monasteries were mostly patriarchal institutions, and even the process of getting ordination as a nun was a Sisyphean task.*

The first Great Retreat had been so successful that Roach and McNally began to plan for a second one to begin at the end of the decade. As they traveled around the world lecturing about their insights into the inner workings of a divine universe, they promised that students who followed them now could study tantra with them in person. After seven years, their most qualified students would be able to lock themselves away in the desert in an updated retreat compound. It would be the second Great Retreat, sometimes also called the Retreat for Peace. They promised that it would save the world.

For Roach, karma wasn't only something that worked over the course of many lives, it was something that could play out in a matter of months, or even days. The couple reduced the calculus of karma to

---

*The Buddha gave nuns 331 vows to adhere to while monks had only 227. Most original nun lineages back to the Buddha died out in the 1400s, but there has been a concerted effort among Buddhist groups around the world to revive them. In 2005 the Dalai Lama gave a speech in Dharamsala to modernize the ordination practice and allow nuns equal access to the tradition, but many women in the ranks still complain that they don't have the same privileges that men do.

a couple of straightforward principles. They held that the surest way to find true love in this life was to give love to a lonely person, and then your ideal lover would simply walk through the door. If you suffer from a chronic illness, the best way to get better is to help someone recover from their own sickness. To achieve great wealth, all you had to do was help someone succeed in their own business affairs. Roach's view of karma unhooked cause from effect and asked his students to see themselves as the cause of their own good and bad fortune, based on intentions alone.

The message was almost irresistible for the superwealthy, who discovered that their good fortune in this life was a sign of a karmic blessing. One of Roach's most notable recruits was Michael Gordon, the founder of a global beauty product line called Bumble and Bumble. Born in England, Gordon was the sort of hairstylist who liked to dream big, and over the course of thirty years his empire grew from a single salon in South Africa into one of the most recognizable hair care brands in the world. The company grossed $50 million in annual sales. Gordon sold his stake in the company in 2006 for $30 million. Afterward, Gordon turned his attention to spiritual matters and donated money for Roach to give a series of lectures on the teachings of Je Tsongkhapa at the Jivamukti Yoga School in New York.

Later, he, Roach, and McNally authored a book together, *Karmic Management: What Goes Around Comes Around in Your Business and Your Life*, laying out principles that would guarantee financial success.

In its introduction, Gordon wrote, "I got into Karmic Management through the back door; once I learned about it I looked back on my business career and realized that it was exactly what I had been doing all along, and why we've been so successful." Gordon credited his rapid accumulation of wealth to a single karmic moment when he felt a strong emotional connection with his first employee—a black woman whom he had hired as a maid at his salon.

In a Herculean effort of noblesse oblige, he decided to teach her how to wash hair like a professional. His first act of charity was to lay his hand on her scalp and scrub her hair himself. "Somewhere inside me," Gordon wrote in *Karmic Management*, "I feel that this small act to help the world is what really sowed the seed for Bumble's future success." The experience of teaching skills to a woman who was far below his station and on the other side of a racial divide stuck with Gordon. It became a totem of his own capacity for humility, which offered him a way to conceive of the success of Bumble and Bumble's aggressive expansion across world markets. Bumble and Bumble was successful because Gordon himself was a good person—the universe organized itself around his own feelings and intentions. Roach, McNally, and Gordon started lecturing together and put up a website to advertise the ideas behind karmic management.

The rich, it turned out, were looking for a philosophy like this. Soon an oil conglomerate director in Kiev asked Roach and McNally to teach him their methods. Donations flowed back to ACI and they used the chance to fund-raise more money for constructing buildings at Diamond Mountain.

Though his karma may have felt clear, in 2012 the IRS arrested Gordon on charges of tax fraud. According to the criminal complaint, an inside source who worked closely with Gordon over the years alleged that during the time that he was helping write the book on karmic management, Gordon was also "actively seeking ways to hide money from the IRS, including sending money overseas, so that he would not have to pay taxes on that income." Indeed, rather than pay his share, Gordon filed a tax return requesting $39,000 back from the government. Though the case continues to wind its way through bail hearings and back-door appeals, just weeks after the arrest, the karmic management website quietly disappeared from the Internet, as did many records of Roach's public affiliations with Gordon.*

When Ian Thorson moved to Germany with Beatrice Steimer, it seemed like a new era of tranquility had begun. He lost himself in Steimer and they lived together in a small railroad apartment. It was

---

*According to Jigme Palmo, a Diamond Mountain board member, "Roach and Gordon were never very close. Roach has been liberal with sharing bylines with people who perhaps don't really deserve the credit."

a concrete slab building in the old Jewish quarter near museums and galleries that was perhaps a little nicer than the ones around it. In a few months Steimer would bear their baby girl, and Thorson threw himself into any job that would offer him a living wage. A family connection scored him a gig translating academic books into English. Some days he strapped on a tie over a rumpled shirt and made his way to part of the city thick with glass-and-steel sky-rises where he had a job tutoring business executives who wanted to improve their English. Stephen Lindberg, who hired Ian to research a book, remembered that Ian was shy about mentioning anything with a Buddhist connection. The couple continued to drive to the occasional meditation retreat, but Ian tried to keep that part of his life secret from his family back home. Thea Steimer was born in November 2001 with a mop of wavy black hair on her head.

After a year, Ian wrote a letter to his former girlfriend Fernanda Hannah, attempting to explain how he had let meditation take up all the space in his life.

> I was using discipline and meditation to get me to a place I did not want to go at all. . . . So I've been taking some time to check out why I started to meditate in the first place. [I wanted] to get closer to others, not further and I do not think I will go back to it until I figure how I went wrong and how to correct it. I can't explain much more, but Buddhism and my teachers are all good but what I was doing with it was off without really knowing it. I was using the meditation to get some kind of good feeling not to get closer to others. It was really tricky to notice it, to catch myself getting into some kind of good feeling, even in conversations with other people. To do what I was doing was not at all Buddhism, but me just being selfish.
>
> —Ian Thorson, January 2001

Their relationship rekindled over e-mail, letters, and phone calls and they lamented that it was difficult to see each other from across the Atlantic.

It wasn't until 2003, when Roach was out of retreat and he and McNally made a stopover in Berlin, that the aura of stability began to crack. Bumble and Bumble had arranged a series of lectures there and helped by using their connections to pack an audience hall, including reaching out to Steimer to translate. Ian hadn't seen Roach for years, but he drank in the teachings like water in a desert. When they had a chance to meet in private, Christie McNally saw Ian's elation and asked him to come back to Arizona and film the construction of a new Diamond Mountain campus. She and Roach planned to compile an online course pack and videotape all of their lectures, and they needed his help. It was the age of e-dharma, and students would be able to download teachings for free: Millions of people would listen to the lectures and have their lives changed for the better.

McNally enticed him further with the whiff of new tantric teachings. With the Great Retreat over, she and Roach had begun to draw on a fresh repository of secret knowledge. It was a tempting offer, but Steimer wasn't interested in uprooting again. Money was tight, and success hadn't come to Ian as easily as he felt he deserved it. The meeting sent Ian back into a tailspin. It was so much easier for him to search for the world he wanted to see, not the one he was living in.

Soon after Ian reconnected with Roach, Fernanda landed an internship with a major architecture firm in Barcelona. When her company offered her a chance to look at a factory in Berlin, she arranged to meet Ian between appointments. She was excited to see how parenthood had changed him. They decided to meet at a museum. Crowds of people passed by the corner where Fernanda waited as she scanned all of their faces, waiting for a spark of recognition. From out of the crowd Ian emerged pushing a baby stroller. She rushed to hug her once-lover and bent down to grab Thea, but when she looked at the infant, the excitement drained from her face. The child was filthy; her clothes looked matted and gray as if she had been wearing the same onesie for a week. It was the sort of filth that might cause bedsores.

In New York she knew that Ian had sometimes eschewed washing, but now she yelled at him that "the same thing shouldn't apply to Thea." Ian shrugged in response. Parenthood had made things between Beatrice and him more difficult, and he sheepishly admitted that the day care program Thea attended sent her home on a few occasions because she was too dirty. Fernanda went home wondering if she would ever see him again, and if she did, who Ian would turn out to be.

Ian, it seemed, was going through another metamorphosis. He was more agitated than he had ever been before. Beatrice said that when he got angry he had a tendency to take his aggression out on the things in her apartment, throwing glasses and bashing his hand against walls.

Reconnecting with McNally and Roach put Thorson back in touch with the vast network of students who signed up for courses through the Asian Classics Institute website. The apartment in Berlin became a hub for ACI students passing through Germany. When they showed up, Ian benevolently rolled out mattresses for the guests and lent them keys.

In 2004, Deborah Bye, a slight, stringy-blond barrister from Australia, connected with Ian through her yoga instructor. The weekend was a busy one, and Ian had plans for a trip out into the country with Beatrice and Thea, so he said Bye could have the apartment to herself for a few days. It was a generous offer and Bye entertained herself around town, meeting friends for coffee and cake and coming back late in the evening.

One night when Bye returned, the lights were on in the house. As she worked her key in the lock, Ian heard the noise, sprang to his feet, and threw open the door. Not knowing what was wrong, Bye stood there in shock while Ian yelled for her to get out. The rage seethed off of him, his face red, his eyes glistening. She started to pack her bags, but Ian was relentless. He grabbed a suitcase and threw it out into the hall. She begged him not to rush her, but he just kept charging.

Thea cried in the background as Ian grabbed Deborah by the hair and pulled the older woman to the top of the steep flight of stairs. Afraid that he might kick her, she covered her head and hunkered on the ground. "I was screaming in terror. I did not know what he was going to do. I felt he might kill me," she wrote later in a report that she filed with the Berlin police. "It was just as if he snapped suddenly without warning," she wrote. Ian tossed the suitcase out the door and it struck Deborah on her back, leaving her with a deep purple bruise.

Deborah Bye left Berlin the following night, unable to comprehend the sudden turn of violence. Beatrice refused to speak about the incident, so it is hard to know exactly what sparked the change in Ian's personality, except that it appears that life in Berlin was not as simple as he had envisioned. The perfect world that he imagined didn't square with the one where a parent needs to clean up endless soiled diapers.

What is clear, however, is that the conflict was a catalyst that made Steimer ask Thorson to move out. Before Bye decided to file her police report, Ian was already planning to head back to Diamond Mountain. McNally's offer for him to help craft the future of dharma in America was simply too enticing. He was failing as a parent and as a partner. Perhaps Diamond Mountain was the only place that would still have him and the only place where he might be able to make sense out of his life.

After he returned to America, records of Ian's life begin to disappear. It is as if the sudden surge of violent tendencies erased his will to record his thoughts. No longer interested in talking with his family or friends from his past, Ian simply stopped writing. His own story began to merge into the landscape and constant flow of people around Diamond Mountain. Ian was just one face in a wave of volunteers who answered the call Roach and McNally broadcasted on their lecture tour and convened in Arizona. Investment bankers, nurses, lawyers, real estate moguls, musicians, and construction workers took time off from their jobs to volunteer to construct a series of yurts, houses, and temples that would one day become the permanent foundation for Diamond Mountain.

At first it wasn't much to look at, but the builders had a vision. Two valleys cut the retreat grounds in half. Closest to the entrance would be a few small yurts and a trailer park for welcoming occasional visitors. Next to the parking lot a one-story building served as a temple for the various ceremonies and events that the group put on.

Behind the temple, students placed offerings of dark chocolate, gemstones, and trinkets on a large, white stucco, Tibetan-style stupa. Across the dirt road, a kitchen and office space called Jamyang House held supplies and an industrial freezer, as well as the administrative offices where the day-to-day work got done. In their spare time, volunteers planted a small garden and arranged a seating area where they could relax during their brief moments of respite. The entrance valley was open to the public, but it was far from the heart of activity.

Higher up on the hill was the Lama House, where Roach stayed with McNally when they were in town. The dirt road that cuts through the property forks a quarter mile from the kitchens: To the right is the entrance that park rangers use to access the administrative offices of Fort Bowie; to the left a locked gate with two cowboy boots nailed on top of its fence posts guards the entrance to the retreat valley itself.

McNally wanted a second Great Retreat to be more ambitious than the last one. Instead of only a couple of humble yurts on a desolate property, the retreat near Fort Bowie would have dozens of highly efficient solar-powered and self-cooling structures. The permanent infrastructure on Diamond Mountain property could host scores of retreatants over long periods of time, with a steady staff of volunteers living down below who vowed to take care of the meditators' every need. Roach and McNally planned to lead forty people into the desert on a quest to see emptiness directly. They had no problem finding followers to foot the bill.

To finance the construction, McNally asked every prospective retreatant to build and pay for their own retreat cabin. When the retreat was over, ownership of the cabins would revert to Diamond Mountain as a donation. The most modestly priced cabin cost around $10,000 for a mud yurt whose dome resembled something that Luke Skywalker would recognize from the surface of Tatooine. More lavish retreat spaces hovered closer to $300,000 for a veritable paradise. Volunteers like Ian, along with a few professional contractors, labored for several years on the designs while Roach and McNally prepped the spiritual seekers with philosophy and new meditation techniques.

Fifteen miles down the dirt road from Diamond Mountain is the small town of Bowie. Once a bastion for the tourism trade, today much of the city is in a preserved state of decay. Abandoned hotels covered with graffiti wilt on their foundations. A significant segment of the population survives in trailer homes as if they might take up and leave at any moment. Here, Michael Brannan's trailer sits next to a cinder-block convenience store that seems to sell only Mexican beer. Sitting at a small foldout table next to an altar stuffed with pictures of Michael Roach wearing a blindfold during the first retreat teachings, and another photo of the Dalai Lama, Brannan cracks open a beer and stuffs a slice of lime inside.

Brannan is fifty-one and has long hair and leathery skin from working in the sun. He puffs out his chest with pride when he says that he was one of the first people to volunteer to build the retreat yurts. He began following Roach at the beginning of the millennium and spent almost seven years as a full-time volunteer. Drawn to complex philosophical discussions, Brannan took on a role leading Buddhist debates among the students. During debates, students lined up in long rows and barked Tibetan philosophy at one another, occasionally clapping their hands and shouting to make a point. It's an old tradition that dates back to monasteries in Tibet and allows students to hone their command of the dharma. Brannan's job was to be sure that the students' arguments adhered to Buddhist logic.

Now that he no longer goes to Diamond Mountain regularly, he feels conflicted about his teacher. On one hand he loves the way that Buddhism orders the universe, but he also worries that Roach is so absorbed by his own spiritual progress that he forgets the world around him. "I got two years of good sutra teachings before Geshe Michael began focusing on tantra. I'm thankful for that," Brannan says with a genuine smile.

The switch to teaching tantra troubled Brannan as debates started to focus less on how to make the world a better place and more on how to take individuals closer to enlightenment. Roach's emergence with McNally on his arm made Brannan question Roach's judgment. McNally never held a job of her own outside of Roach's organization, and though she had a myriad of responsibilities within the group, it is easy to see how she was getting in over her head. "He called her Vajrayogini! Can you imagine being promoted to goddess by your husband and guru?" asks Brannan.

More important, when McNally spoke, the teachings were diluted, as if Roach was stepping back. "I used to think that sometimes he just had a dazed look in his eyes when she gave talks," says Brannan.

And yet, most students liked the more experiential focus of tantra over the more brooding sutras. Sid Johnson, a long-haired musician from Canada who arrived in Bowie with his wife, also fell out with the group. Though he came simply to study philosophy for free, he proved to be competent and had a flexible enough schedule that Roach asked him to join the Diamond Mountain board of directors. Johnson helped build the original campus at St. David and could help advise the volunteers on the ongoing construction. He didn't always consider himself a Buddhist, but enjoyed the company, and liked experimenting with the techniques that he hoped might help him live a fuller life.

In 2005, Johnson sat in a packed audience hall with Roach and McNally on the stage. The topic of the day was guru devotion—the couple's devotion to each other was obvious—but at times it was difficult for students to wrap their minds around the idea that every command a guru offered was a potential teaching moment. Roach exclaimed that since taking McNally as his spiritual partner, she was also his lama and he would do anything she asked. "Such as if Christie asked him to stab himself with a knife, he would do it without hesitation," recalls Johnson, paraphrasing the lecture. At those words, Roach jumped up and retrieved a small ritual dagger from the altar and jammed it into his hand. "He stabbed himself really hard! Christie screamed 'NO!' and we all sat up as she pulled it from his hand. Roach starts whimpering and crying and she comforted him." It was all very theatrical and staged, but the blood was real. Students who were in awe of the couple for the example they set puzzled about the event for weeks. Do you harm yourself if your lama asks it of you? What are the limits of unconditional surrender? Johnson chalked it up to an adolescent game gone awry. Other people were not so sure.

In general, the ceremonies on Diamond Mountain leaned toward the dramatic. It was a type of showmanship that is all but absent in the more reserved monasteries in India. Even the one where Khen Rinpoche taught in New Jersey had a more reserved air, more like a Latin mass than a Baptist revival. Initiations that might take an afternoon of recitations in a Tibetan monastery in Dharamsala morphed into showpieces designed to elicit emotional responses. Roach wanted his students to feel the dharma, not just understand it. And the secrecy around tantra made it all the more exciting.

Shortly after Roach stabbed himself in the hand, Johnson took an initiation with eighty other people for the bull-headed Buddhist tantric deity Yamantaka. The deity's name translates literally into the "defeater of death."

The ritual stretched across four days, and every day senior students, mostly women who had been on the first three-year retreat, gave separate teachings. The event culminated with every student taking a private ceremony with Geshe Michael and Lama Christie in which they earned the final empowerment meant to conquer death. Johnson was nervous when he entered the room wearing a blindfold. Geshe Michael asked him to lie down on their bed. He did so and then Roach and Christie started massaging his chakras, starting with his head and ending at his penis. "I'm not sure who undid my pants, but it was part of the blessing," Johnson remembers. When they were done, he sat up—still wearing a blindfold—and felt McNally's lips press against his. They began to kiss. "There is part of the initiation where your lama is supposed to give you his consort, and the way Geshe Michael teaches it, the things that happen in the metaphysical world also have to happen in the real one," says Johnson. When they were finished, they giggled like children at a summer camp breaking taboos and no one else would know. Ten minutes later they asked Johnson's wife to come in alone.

Allison Dey also volunteered at Diamond Mountain and, like Johnson, had spent more than ten years working with Roach and McNally. She studied tantra with Roach but tended to prefer imagining a spiritual angel as her partner rather than interacting with a real person during meditation. It was a valid method; in fact it was the one that orthodox Tibetans teach in lieu of partner practice. But it wasn't the sort of meditation Roach emphasized. "I was a lucky one where I didn't have to get called into a weird situation," she remembers, "before I really knew anything about tantra. I knew that it was possible that there would be deep practices where your teacher might get you into the room alone. What ends up being a sexual-looking practice is designed to move your inner winds." Even so, she said she would have been open to the possibility if it took her further down the spiritual path.

Partner practice seemed to have its pitfalls even for Roach and McNally. As a shortcut toward enlightenment, it pushed students to embrace complex parts of their own psyches, but the implications of visualization had a tendency to spill over into real life. McNally and Roach meditated on their perfect angelic partners during sexual union. McNally visualized Roach as her perfect angel. It turned out that Roach let his mind wander. He focused his on "other women that he saw as Angels," she recalled later in an interview with Nina Burleigh, reporting for *Rolling Stone*. According to Dey and other sources who overheard the couple's squabbles, Roach contemplated the girlfriend he'd dated when he was sixteen years old.* At least one source states that it was the same woman who had caused an outcry among the clergy in Howell, New Jersey, when Roach tried to put her face on a book titled *Preparing for Tantra*. Other sources recounted a string of lovers on the side, whom Roach dubbed as angels, at least for short sessions. How that might have worked with McNally and him only fifteen feet apart stretches the imagination.

Roach wanted to make the real world appear more like the one in his visions. At the temple in the lower valley, the board of Diamond Mountain threw parties called *tsechus* awash in ritually blessed alcohol, and encouraged students to break social taboos. According to Ekan Thomason, who enrolled in the tantric courses, Roach sometimes showed up in drag. "He was dressed like a preppy girl in a skirt," she remembered. In his worship of the goddess, Roach hoped to get in touch with his feminine side and encouraged other men to do the same. Following his lead, Thomason ordered Roach a gift of women's underwear from a Japanese website that catered to crossdressers. It was specially designed to accommodate the male bulge.

The contrasting images of Roach—one as a conservative and authentic monk on the lecture circuit, and the other as a cross-dressing rule breaker—encouraged new students to embrace contradictions

---

*The woman in question refused a request to speak on or off the record.

in religious teachings. As pupils strove to attain more exclusive knowledge, the taboo-breaking drove some people away from Diamond Mountain. Those who stayed felt as if they were in a secret club and they could bond over the illicitness.

While Roach could explain his peculiar spiritual path to students, without a ringing endorsement from the Dalai Lama there would always be questions about whether what he taught really was Buddhism and not an inspired offshoot. So Roach planned to court the Dalai Lama's blessing by traveling back to India and teaching on His Holiness's home turf in the Himalayan town of Dharamsala.

The Dalai Lama's annual speech attracts tens of thousands of Buddhist practitioners. Typically he lectures in high Tibetan, which only the most learned foreigners can make out. Instead, attendees tune in to his speeches on small transistor radios where UN-style translators deliver His Holiness's teachings in a variety of world languages. Roach's appeal had long been his adeptness at speaking the dharma directly in English, so he scheduled a talk at the Tibetan Institute of Performing Arts about a mile above the site where the Dalai Lama would speak. The schedule was similar to the one that he employed in Bodh Gaya at the turn of the millennium. It was the sort of affront that should be inexcusable, like a member of Congress preempting the U.S. president's State of the Union address.

The plan failed dramatically. One source reports that the Dalai Lama was drinking a cup of tea when he heard the news. The cup shook in his fingers, and both the cup and the saucer he was holding clattered to the floor. Before Roach even arrived in India, the Dalai Lama's office issued a public letter that banned him from setting foot in Dharamsala. The letter was addressed to Reverend Roach, a slight that was considerably below Roach's academic qualification and seemed to put the very validity of his geshe degree into question.

More to the point, the office requested that Roach prove his spiritual realizations.

If you have reached the path of seeing, as you claim in your letter, you should then be able to show extraordinary powers and perform miracles

like the Siddhas of the past. Only then will the followers of Tibetan
Buddhists be able to believe and accept your claims.

—Tenzin Geyche Tethong, Secretary to H. H.

The Dalai Lama, May 24, 2006

Though neither Roach nor McNally ever performed any miracles in public, various students at Diamond Mountain claimed to have had supernatural experiences with the couple. A member, who asked to remain anonymous, said she saw Roach and McNally at one *tsechu* walk through a wall of the temple building by bending the laws of space and time. She stood there with her mouth hanging wide open. McNally gave her a secret smile and handed her a baseball hat with the ACI logo on it.

In another account, Sid Johnson remembers that when he was picking up supplies for Diamond Mountain in Tucson, he parked his battered pickup truck on a hill and walked away. When he turned around he saw that the emergency brake had failed and the truck was rolling away from him out of control. It careened toward a busy intersection, when out of nowhere a person appeared in front of the truck and stopped it with his bare hands. Johnson watched slack-jawed as the man—or apparition—pushed the heavily loaded vehicle back up the hill to its old spot and then walked away without saying a word.

Johnson and other sources who witnessed the supposed miracles are critical of many things that happened on Diamond Mountain, but they also can't find any other way to explain their experiences. Was it a divine intervention, or were their minds playing tricks on them? Diana Alstad, the coauthor with Joel Kramer of *The Guru Papers*, explains the phenomenon of these perceived miracles on a psychological level. "People can convince themselves that they have seen many things that are really just projections of their own mind." She says that disciples give their mental energy to a guru, and the guru returns the energy to their followers, not unlike what happens at a great rock concert where the band and crowd feed on each other's energy. Only with a guru, that energy gets read in spiritual, and sometimes miraculous, terms.

The explanation is comforting, but thinking of such stories simply as hallucinations isn't straightforward either. Sid Johnson doubts the validity of Roach's philosophy but doesn't question his own experiences: "I don't know what to say other than it was a miracle." The original *Yoga Sutras of Patanjali* openly state that such things are possible with intense devotion but that cultivating powers does not make someone innately closer to ultimate truth. Even if Roach could walk through a wall, or stop a traffic accident in progress, does it necessarily mean he was perfect in other ways?

Powers or no, Alstad believes that McNally's proximity to Roach altered her in profound and possibly permanent ways: "Roach took her mind over, or she gave it to him. That is what a follower does: They surrender."

But McNally's surrender could last only until Roach's own spiritual aspirations began to impinge on his commitment to her. When Roach meditated on women other than his wife—the woman he publicly declared a goddess—he undermined the eternal love that the two wanted to project. It was one contradiction too far.

By 2009, as the final plans for the second Great Retreat were under way, McNally had had enough. In her interview with *Rolling Stone*, she explained that she told Roach, "'Listen, I can't do this anymore. Either be a faithful partner to me, like you are claiming—in body, speech, AND mind—or I will start behaving the same way you do.' His response was that this was the situation I had walked into, and he had no intention of changing. Long story short, he started moving away from me and pushing me towards Ian."

They broke up and the fallout from the split reverberated through the community. Some students teared up as if their parents had divorced. Ekan Thomason originally planned to go on the second Great Retreat and, under McNally's direction, had built a cabin at her own expense, but watching the couple break up gave her second thoughts. "It was like everything he had been teaching about spiritual partnerships being eternal was torn to pieces," she said. The infidelity rippled through the community and tore apart couples who, from the outside, had looked bedrock-solid. "A lot of people just sort of swapped partners," remembers Michael Brannan. Including, of course, Lama Christie McNally herself.

After Roach spent the better part of twelve years pouring the secrets of his lineage into McNally, he learned that it is a lot easier to make a goddess than it is to unmake one. Faced with the possibility of being stuck in a yurt near his ex-wife for three years, Roach handed McNally the reins of the retreat as if it were a divorce settlement. She would don the mantle of retreat leader while Roach settled for the title of spiritual leader in absentia. The breakup didn't always make sense to disciples who had listened to speeches extolling the possibility of undying love. The shattering of their success story weakened many people's faith. However, since Roach's tantric teachings often emphasized embracing contradictions, some people thought that it was simply another lesson for them to absorb. Allison Dey, one of sixty people who stayed on the land, shrugged. "They were too intense. In my opinion breaking up was good for them."

Far from being turned off by relationships, Roach seemed to take the shuffle of partners in stride—using it as an opportunity to anoint a new cast of members into leadership positions and arranging new spiritual marriages between his followers. Eric Brinkman, an ex-military officer who fell into Roach's orbit in 2003 after he found free videos of Roach's lectures on the web, had spent seven years studying Tibetan logic, tantra, and philosophy. He was ready to extend his commitment to the organization by taking vows to become a monk. At the ceremony that changed Brinkman's name to Nyingpo and his clothing to maroon robes, Roach declared that rather than holding Brinkman to a vow of celibacy, Brinkman needed his own spiritual consort. Roach waved his arm wide and pointed to Mercedes Bahleda, his longtime personal assistant. Roach called Mercedes onto the stage to stand next to the neophyte monk. A dozen or more people in attendance chimed together that "Mercedes and Nyingpo are one!"*

---

*Both Bahleda and Brinkman deny that their partnership began in this way. Bahleda wrote to me in an e-mail, "No this never happened and is a complete fabrication. Many people who attended will know your book is false if you write this. No one in the audience said anything that I heard, nor was asked to [sic], what you have written below made me laugh. Geshe Michael Roach merely conducted a monk's ordination; he never mentioned anything about a partnership."

Ian and Christie

Let's not be shy. The goal of our spiritual practice is to reach a state of
pure bliss. You can call it heaven if you like, or enlightenment, or
liberation. But we are talking about constant unbridled elation.
— Lama Christie McNally and Ian Thorson,
Two As One: A Journey to Yoga

THE SMALL WOODEN SKIFF set a parallel course to the white sand
beach. The outboard motor cut through the meditative peace cherished by the owners of the resort and announced the arrival of Lama
Christie McNally and Ian Thorson. A wooden sign with bright yellow painted letters hanging above the dock read SIVANANDA RETREAT
CENTER.

The wellness institution in the heart of the Bahamas draws an
international clientele that is eager to absorb lessons on Ayurveda,
yoga, sacred art, and meditation. Founded in the tradition of a popular Hindu mystic who helped bring yoga to the West, the center
blends sacred New Age thought with exotic Caribbean vacations.
People here are young, hip, often wealthy, and beautiful. Vacationers
sign up for beachside yoga classes and sip carefully prepared fruit-
and-herb concoctions designed to balance their energies. Ian and
Christie came here to give a lecture together on the possibility of
eternal love, the necessity for meditation, and how people could use
yoga to strengthen the bonds of their relationship. In the mornings
during their stay, and like every morning since they got together,

McNally and Thorson meditated facing each other, their gazes fixed on the foreverness hidden in each other's eyes. As they warmed up, the routine morphed into an idiosyncratic yoga invented to bring couples closer together. In it, they pulled on each other's limbs and used their own body weight to gracefully deepen their partner's pose. They wore matching necklaces featuring silver infinity signs tightly around their necks, and both had diamond studs in their ears. It was as if McNally was reliving her relationship with Roach, except this time she was the guru.

On one afternoon, they decided they would take a walk together in one of the teeming jungles on a nearby island. They engaged a skiff and motored across the crystal blue waters, where the captain dropped them off and left them alone to walk into the forest. Brightly colored kingfishers and parrots flitted across the canopy, and feral pigs rooted along the beach. Ripe tamarind hung heavily from the tree stalks like jackfruit, and coconuts ballooned off the tops of palm trees. As they meandered into nature with no particular object in mind, a tawny dog followed in their footsteps. It was the type of animal that hangs around people, looking for scraps, neither wild nor tame but happy to exist on what people give it. It begged with its eyes, as dogs do.

Time passed and the path grew convoluted. They knew they had time to eventually reach the dock to catch the boat back to Nassau Island, where the retreat was, but every path they took seemed to lead them farther away from their bearings. They wandered, and the sun arced across the sky toward dusk. Ian tried to lead but was confounded at every juncture. Christie was not as sure-footed in nature as Ian, but she trusted her partner to set things right.

He worried that they would have to spend the night alone in the jungle, where they would be bitten by mosquitoes and forced to endure the elements rather than enjoying each other's company in a tropical paradise. They hadn't packed much food, and as it got later, they felt the tidings of fear. The dog had followed them for much of the day, but as night drew near, it decided that there would be no more treats forthcoming and trotted off in the direction opposite to where they had been traveling. Lacking any other ideas, Ian suggested that they follow the animal.

With its intimate knowledge of its home island, the dog had no trouble finding its way. It was not lost. Within a half hour they were back by the dock, and the boatman was ready to take them back to the spa. Had the dog never followed them, Ian and Christie could have ended up scared and alone at night. Thorson took it as a sign. In its own way, the dog was a guardian angel—a guide out of darkness.

For five years Ian had blended into the fabric of daily life at Diamond Mountain. Since returning from Germany, he barely had contact with his family in New York and instead threw himself into every practice prescribed by his two lamas. Without interference from the outside, he could enter into meditative states for days at a time or explore the arid hills around Fort Bowie. Most notably, he was often at the lamas' cabin—on hand for whatever errand McNally or Roach needed fulfilled.

Within a month of his arrival from Germany he met a bespectacled yogini named Anna Wheeler. Tattoos unraveled down her arms, and one, a striking picture of an Indian woman in traditional dress, gave Wheeler a rebel vibe. She had a master's degree in gender studies from San Francisco State and had fun disassembling underlying notions of patriarchy. Entranced by Ian's natural good looks and philosophical mind, she became pregnant with his second child almost immediately. It was an accident, and the couple was hesitant to make a serious commitment to each other. Roach taught that abortion is a cardinal sin, and there was never any real question about Wheeler not carrying the fetus to term.

Though she saw something special in Thorson, Wheeler had few illusions about his being an attentive father. According to multiple sources, Ian came back from Germany still unable to control the bouts of rage that boiled up from within him. During an argument Ian pushed her against a doorway, sending her to the ground and making her fear for the safety of her child. Wheeler extricated herself from the relationship and gave birth to Ian's son, Deva, at a hospital in New York in 2007.

Thorson had other women—flings mostly—until he paired himself with Nicole Vigna, a massage therapist based in Sonoma's hippie enclave. Vigna was reluctant to admit that Ian exhibited any hints of the violence that had marred his relationships with Steimer and Wheeler. She admired his ability to live without regard for himself and remembers that he was comfortable simply throwing down a blanket and sleeping in one of the washes that run through the sloping canyon. He had no fear of flash floods, roving javelinas, or immigrants who crossed illegally over the land at night. "Ian was a free spirit," she said fondly.

Then, after Roach and McNally split, everything changed. Thorson and Vigna took a car to Ekan Thomason's house outside of the retreat grounds—a small adobe cottage nestled in the imperial rock formation of the Dragoon Mountains. On the way there, the two began to fight. Ian knew whom he wanted as a partner. He dropped Vigna off at Thomason's with just a sleeping bag and a rucksack. He drove down the dirt road to the highway, leaving a thin skein of dust in his wake, and the two women spent the night talking about the abrupt breakup. Vigna seemed confused, saying to Thomason, "Oh, everything is so different, you know. The lamas are not staying together and are going off into their rooms alone." The next time Thomason saw Thorson, he was dancing with McNally at one of the alcohol-fueled parties in the main temple.

The transition to seeing Ian with the goddess sometime in 2010 didn't elicit the sort of gossip that might be typical of a chatty, inwardly focused community. Not everyone liked Ian, but Christie's decision to take him as a partner made a certain sense. He'd spent most of his adult life studying under Roach and had been McNally's personal attendant since he moved to the campus after Germany. Moreover, they looked the part of a loving couple in ways that she never could have with Roach.

Then into his sixties, Roach sported a hairline that had long since receded like the sea at low tide so that the top of his skull was bare and shiny. He liked to joke that he lost his hair stressing over the plight of Tibetan refugees, but standing next to an energetic and ripe woman twenty years his junior, Roach looked like a man in the throes of a midlife crisis reliving his lost youth. Ian was a stark contrast. Lean and corded muscles rippled down his frame—the result of a healthier diet and daily yoga practice. He pulled his dark curly hair back into a ponytail and turned his lips up into a contagious smile. Moreover, in Christie's presence, his near-constant meditation didn't erect a barrier that it had in his relationships with Beatrice and Fernanda. They practiced together. They traveled together. And there was never a problem of Ian having trouble reconciling the meditative world with reality since they both aimed to exist in the same state of mutual bliss. So when McNally suggested that they never stray more than a few feet from each other ever again, it was an easy vow for Thorson to accept.

Later, in an unpublished transcript of an interview by Nina Burleigh in 2013, McNally remembered that while couples typically go through a predictable curve where excitement transformed into comfort and complacency, "This never happened with Ian and myself. There was never any movement away, there was never any feeling of restlessness or boredom, we were each other's favorite thing. Every day was a new discovery of the mystery that was the person next to us. And we were very happy." Their practice and their passion sustained them.

Once inseparable from McNally, Roach seemed to stew at the couple's apparent perfection as any scorned lover might. In one photo from that time, Roach sits on the ground, wearing a shirt printed with the logo SPIRITUAL GANGSTER*; as he watched the duo bend into yoga poses together, the camera caught his face smiling with serene pain. In back rooms with the board of directors of Diamond Mountain, Roach proclaimed that he wouldn't give up control of his spiritual following. Jealous that Thorson might try to usurp some of his

---

*The yoga-wear company Spiritual Gangster was founded by two of Michael Roach's students. It sells "yoga inspired clothing for high vibration living." A woman's cotton tank top with the company logo sells for $45.

authority, Roach tried to pass a measure forbidding board members to discuss administrative matters with partners.

"[We were] uninvited to join Geshe Michael and whatever group he had gathered around him. He made it clear that these were *his* gatherings, and *his* students, and that we should stay away. It got quite uncomfortable for us to even enter the house or to come down-stairs. Eventually Geshe Michael left the house completely and took his gatherings to the house next door. So then students were forced to choose—which house should I go to? We had our gatherings, he had his. Again, very uncomfortable," McNally wrote.*

Whatever was happening behind those closed doors, McNally wasn't just striking out on a new relationship. She was preparing to take her own spiritual practice in new directions. While Roach, how-ever controversially, wore the robes of a Tibetan Buddhist monk, Mc-Nally felt drawn to explore teachings in other traditions.

She knew that the second Great Retreat, which would begin in just over a year's time, would be a proving ground for her as a spiri-tual leader. She may have gained fame by being a vessel for Roach's wisdom, but now she would have to establish her own lineage to be taken seriously in her own right. By the time she finished the second Great Retreat, she would have almost seven years of silent meditation under her belt, a qualification that few Buddhist practitioners—even in Tibet—could claim. Thirty-eight people signed up to walk into the desert with her, and she wanted to impart something special to them. She found her answer outside Tibetan Buddhism in the Hindu god-dess Kali.

The digital archives of the Asian Classics Input Project contain occasional translations of old Hindu initiation rites that made the transition over the Himalayas on the backs of monks. Whether such translations fit with the Tibetan Buddhist orthodoxy is subject to

---

*Board member Nicole Davis clarified in an e-mail: "McNally and Thorson never stopped coming to board meetings. There was a discussion at a board meeting about whether it was appropriate for Ian to come to board meetings since he was not a board member, but no one can dis-invite a board member to a board meeting (and as far as I know, GMR did not dis-invite Christie)."

speculation, but McNally professed that Kali corresponded to the Tibetan goddess Maksurma, or perhaps even Vajrayogini herself.

Kali isn't an ordinary member of the Hindu pantheon. Although a few major temples, including the famous Dakshineswar Kali Temple in Calcutta, are devoted to her worship, most mainstream Hindus invoke her name only in the context of violence or war. At Kalighat, perhaps the most famous temple devoted to the goddess, worshipers sacrifice almost a hundred goats to her every day, their heads severed in a single blow from a sword.* Though her name means "black one," her skin is typically blue and her bloodred tongue arcs sharply down over her chin. Around her neck she wears a garland of human skulls and carries bloodied weapons in seven of her eight hands. Dangling from her last limb is the severed head of one of her foes. More often than not her depictions show her dancing on the corpse of a vanquished god.

In the 1700s, British colonialists popularized and exaggerated stories of Kali worshipers, who were called *Thuggee* (from which we get the English word *thug*). The Thuggee were loosely organized bandits who kidnapped unsuspecting travelers on isolated roads and sacrificed them to the goddess in return for magical powers. The few Hindus who are steeped in tantric practice—usually quite different from Buddhist tantra—will sometimes appeal to Kali for feminine spiritual power, called *shakti*. Sacrifices to the goddess work like contracts: If you offer her something she wants, she grants a boon in return. Though she is willing to accept payment in the form of animal sacrifices, Kali prefers human blood above all other things. In medieval India, history records the names of countless kings who sacrificed children to her before a battle, in return for victory. While she may be untamable, wild, and dangerous, it seems that McNally wanted to add Kali to her tantric meditation to speed her own journey to enlightenment. After all, if Kali could win a war, why couldn't she grant Nirvana too?

---

*Kali, however, does not only accept blood sacrifice. According to Rachel McDermott, a professor at Columbia University, she has seen vegetarian Hindus offer up cucumbers and mangoes to the goddess to sate her thirst—something that, for me, conjures a more benevolent side of the deity: more Bunnicula than Dracula.

In October 2009, McNally took a spot on a throne in a mountain-top building known as the Lama Dome on Diamond Mountain, holding a samurai sword. The squat pink building looked like a cross between an igloo and a yurt and she planned to use it as her living quarters when the retreat began. There, a roomful of prospective initiates had donned special robes and filed into the main chamber. Inside, they found the room decorated with weapons: swords, guns, crossbows, chain saws, and menacing-looking garden implements. Initiates remember being "kidnapped" from their lodgings before the rite and stuffed into a small plywood box to amplify the terror. Ekan Thomason meditated and said the prayers that Lama Christie had asked her to; before she got up from her perch Christie waved a dagger in Thomason's direction.

"Kali requires more of you; she requires your blood," McNally said, reminding Thomason of a beautiful swashbuckling pirate as she ran a finger across the sharp edge of the knife.

The ceremony was designed to be terrifying, and participants were split in their reactions. Some had accepted McNally as an infallible teacher and hoped to learn even in the face of the theatrics. Others worried that Diamond Mountain was losing its way in a turn toward the occult. "I didn't really get it," said Scott Vacek, a board member who accepted the initiation but was baffled by its meaning. The event was divisive and made some of the retreatants worried about what would happen when they locked themselves into the valley with McNally as a leader. Thomason thought the ceremony was a bad omen and withdrew from her spot on the list of retreatants.

Kali added a new dimension to spiritual practice on Diamond Mountain insofar as she allowed a release of pent-up anger and violent energy that wasn't easy to express in the normally tranquil setting. Since most devotees actively tried to live two realities at once—the ordinary world and the extraordinary one—Kali's presence helped create a ritual outlet for the confusion that some people felt when the two worlds clashed. Kali embraced death, destruction, repulsiveness, and decay, and facing her in meditation might help some people come to terms with those aspects of their own existence. For Ian, Kali may have also helped him channel his violent outbursts out of the real world and into the symbolic one, where they wouldn't hurt anyone.

Indeed, that is exactly what seemed to happen. Outside of the tantric world, McNally and Thorson beamed a public face of physical health and perfection. They invented their dynamic version of partner yoga in which they used the weight of the other person's body to deepen their stretches. Then, with the help of the myriad creative people who stalked Diamond Mountain's campus, they produced a remarkable document of their relationship: a book titled *Two As One: A Journey to Yoga*. Printed on heavy glossy paper, it is a compendium of black-and-white photos of Ian and Christie contorting into headstands and back bends and completing their postures with longing gazes. The proceeds of the $25 book went entirely to support the upcoming retreat.

For the shoot, Ian shaved his body, leaving only a thin masculine patch of stubble on his face. From the first page, when the couple bow toward each other in matching black skintight underwear, the ridges of their toned muscles contrast tastefully on the page as they cavort and kiss each other in a loving embrace. Their faces beam joy, not only for each other but for life.

Between pictures of their poses are inspirational passages about the power of yoga to change the world. One passage next to a photo of Ian pulling McNally into a deep back bend stands out from the rest.

> It's not about the pose. It is about that crucial decision of how much trust you give the other person. Then you watch your own mind in its battle between surrender and fear. Your partner is on top of you, smothering you into some forward bend. Are you resisting, are you building a little safety net with your elbows, or can you relax and let them take you as far as you are able to go? Do you push them off when you can't take it anymore, or do you let them decide?
>
> What are we afraid of—a little pain—so what? If you go past pain you'll reach bliss.
>
> Lack of control?
>
> The practice of surrender is Lama practice. For this short time on the mat, your partner becomes for you a Guide. You grant them the power to help you.
>
> Don't be wimpy about this! The more you surrender to your partner, the

more they become for you someone who can lead you exactly where you want to go. This practice is bigger than just the two of you. What you do on your mats together really can ripple out and change the world.

So be brave, and kill your fear, for everyone.

McNally had surrendered to her lover as a divine being before. On the first Great Retreat, which began almost ten years earlier, Roach proclaimed that she was an incarnation of Vajrayogini. Now she could be the same thing for Thorson. Their relationship was both divine and physical, and along the way they would experience bliss. When they surrendered to each other they aimed to discover and accept the darkest corners of the other person's psyche. No matter what, they vowed they would be unafraid of what they discovered.

Despite their pending divorce, McNally and Roach still regularly got up on stage together to co-teach the completion of the seven-year course in tantra that was the final qualification before the group was ready to begin their three-year retreat. Ekan Thomason remembers one particularly tense night when the community watched the ex-duo on stage talk about what they might expect on their journeys. Looking out over his flock, Roach asked a rhetorical question:

"Which one of the retreatants do you think will tear off their clothes and run naked through the retreat valley? There is always someone that dies and someone that goes crazy during a three-year retreat," he said. The comment mostly went unmentioned by the audience, but Thomason took note. A few weeks later, in a follow-up class, McNally arrived in the auditorium in her white robes and waited for Roach to meet her. She took her seat on the stage, expecting her lama to show up any minute. The room waited in silence and time slowly ticked by. An hour later a messenger delivered the news that Roach had been "advised by his angel" to skip the lecture. McNally taught the class on her own that night, no doubt wondering who Roach's new angel was.

Whoever it was, Christie was itching to leave the marriage behind her. After she and Ian returned from the Caribbean, they continued their book tour across the world—selling copies at upscale yoga studios from Manhattan to Japan. The tour doubled as an opportunity to say good-bye to friends whom they would not be able to connect with while on retreat. No one was surprised when the tour also turned into an announcement that they were going to formalize their commitment in marriage. They hatched a hasty plan to get hitched near where Ian had grown up surfing in the ritzy New York vacation town of Montauk.

There was only one legal hurdle to overcome. Though their relationship went public after the first Great Retreat, almost no one knew that Roach and McNally had actually legally married at a secret ceremony in Little Compton, Rhode Island. The legal aspect of their split had never been resolved. So in advance of the wedding in Montauk, McNally urged her ex-lover to file the official divorce paperwork in a Yavapai County courthouse. The agreement gave McNally custody of the couple's red Dodge Durango, and Roach, a small house in Rimrock, Arizona, where he might one day retire. It divided copyrights of their various books, and allowed Roach to finish a book they had planned to write together—the forthcoming *Karma of Love,* which was meant to answer the one hundred most common questions that keep couples apart. McNally relinquished her right to work on the book and let him finish it on his own.*

As they hastily prepared for their wedding day the couple stayed on Roosevelt Island with Ian's family. It was an odd arrangement but one that Kay found promising as a time to reconnect with her lost son. Ian used his time in New York to meet up with his long-lost Stanford friend Saul Kato. In the intervening years, Kato had followed the path of a Stanford tech baron. He set up and sold several tech startups at a profit, and went on to earn an advanced degree in neuroscience. They'd lost touch completely after Ian went to Germany, but the invitation to the marriage gave them an excuse to get together.

Kato smiled broadly when he remembered how Ian showed up with Christie in her white robes. "Ian liked a challenge. It did not surprise me at all that he stole the cult leader's main squeeze."

---

*According to the divorce records, McNally and Roach filed for a separation on September 21, 2010, just two weeks before McNally and Thorson's wedding in Montauk. The papers were finalized by the court on December 1, 2010, meaning that Thorson and McNally's marriage may not have had legal standing.

For Kato, it seemed a sort of sophomoric accomplishment, but he also saw that the upcoming retreat might be an opportunity to advance the field of neuroscience. Kato wondered how three years of silence and meditation might change his friend's brain and asked Ian to sit in an MRI scanner to analyze what the neurology of enlightenment might look like. Assuming he was successful, were there any specific sorts of brain changes that correspond to high realizations? Ian got excited at the prospect and rushed home to his mother to tell her about it.

The project was ambitious and its logistics were daunting. To get scanned during the retreat meant that Ian would have to take a break for a few days and travel to Tucson, and McNally warned that the interruption would disturb his practice and that leaving the retreat for the real world for even a few hours would be a bad idea. So the brain scan idea never took hold. "It's too bad that it didn't happen," remembered Kato when I met him at a research institute outside of San Diego. "We might have really learned what was going on in his mind." Kay Thorson remains disappointed to this day. She hoped that Ian would have used the experiment to help further science, and perhaps explain the neurological basis for Ian's drive toward the divine.

A week or two later, some of Ian's family came together and traveled out to Montauk. It was a surprisingly traditional affair. McNally wore a white wedding dress with a lacy veil that cascaded down over her right eye and a double strand of pearls that hung lightly on her neck. They stood on a bluff by the sea, and a priest read them their vows. Roach wasn't there, but about a hundred guests witnessed their commitment. The bridesmaids wore blue to the wedding, but Alexandra Thorson, Ian's sister, declined the invitation to attend. She couldn't bring herself to care anymore about his next steps. Though she hoped he was happy, she knew that her brother was gone once and for all. "Well, they got married, and then their honeymoon was to go on this three-year silent retreat," she said. "That was pretty much the end of it for me. It was just over at that point for me."

When the ceremony was over, the guests returned to their homes. The newlyweds left for Diamond Mountain for the first and last time as a couple.

12.

Exodus

How can it be an accident when my hand was the one holding the knife?
—Lama Christie McNally

WINTER STRUCK THE Arizona desert like a hammer. On the last
night of December 2011, Lama Christie and thirty-nine retreatants
gathered together in the temple building with their friends and families. Strong winds funneled through the mountain valley and kicked
up dust and debris. People had come from all over the world: British
citizens, Australians, Israelis, but most of the retreatants were Americans. Even though the room was cramped with bodies, their combined heat wasn't enough to allow them to shuck their winter coats.
Some rubbed the arms of their jackets to keep warm; others just
smiled and shivered beneath their frocks. The barriers of the retreat
were set, the cabins built, and McNally had whittled down the final
list of lock-ins, from a hundred folks who said they were ready to take
on the commitment to only those most dedicated to the mission. The
night had a bittersweet air to it: It was the last moment any of the retreatants would see their families for a thousand days. They knew the
world would go on without them, that they would lose friends and
abandon lovers. Some must have wondered if it would be worth it.

Christie McNally climbed to the stage to offer her farewell speech. Her task was not simple. She had to convince them that the commitment was not just a solipsistic enterprise to delve into the roots of their own psyches but an earnest attempt to save the world. The yurts were laboratories, and the retreatants, scientists of the same order as the men who designed the atom bomb. Together the group would unlock the fundamental laws of the universe. In three years some of them would emerge as Bodhisattvas.

Some people in the audience who had come to see their friends off had no background in Buddhism. So to explain what they were doing, McNally began to recount the plot of the movie *The Matrix*. In the film a young Keanu Reeves plays Neo, a computer programmer who accidentally discovers that the world he lives in—that all of us live in—is actually a simulation run on computer servers the size of skyscrapers. The real world is a desolate postapocalyptic hellscape where humans are mostly enslaved to machines. After Neo discovers the true nature of the computer program that runs the world, he realizes that he can change the code to obey his will. He stops time, bends spoons with his mind, and flies through a crowded cityscape like Superman. All the while, the forces that have a stake in maintaining the illusion—personified by black suit–wearing G-men—pursue him at every turn. For McNally, *The Matrix* was a perfect metaphor.

I was trying to figure out how I'm going to tell you about emptiness. That's pretty close. We were actually really amazed that they made a movie about us! . . . That's what we are trying to do. All the ancient texts that we have been studying for the past six years have been telling us how our world is not what it seems. How everything around us in our reality is not really out there in the way that we think it is. It is coming from somewhere else. It is coming from seeds inside of our own heart. It is like a virtual reality that is being projected out, but it is not some über-computer that is projecting it, it is us. We are the ones projecting our reality. And there are a lot of amazing implications from that. It means that you could do what Neo did. Then anything in the world that you don't like you could just reach inside your own heart and change a few

things and then the world would change. And we are here in the three-
year retreat to see if we can do that.
—Lama Christie's Talk to Retreatants' Families, December 2010

Retreat coordinators recorded the evening on video. A salt-and-pepper-haired Scott Vacek scanned his camera over the audience and asked McNally to make one last video pitch for donations. Since they began fund-raising, the Diamond Mountain board had amassed almost $1.5 million in donations, speaking fees by McNally and Roach, as well as the meager royalties from their books. It was enough to own the land beneath their feet, but keeping the retreat running was still in question. McNally pleaded with the unseen audience to donate a dollar a day to sustain them and allow the volunteers in the base camp to keep their kitchens stocked with wholesome meals.

The second Great Retreat was an industrial-size version of the first one: a sort of enlightenment factory. They called it the Retreat for Peace, and if all went according to plan, Diamond Mountain would grow into one of the most important centers for Tibetan Buddhist meditation in the Western Hemisphere. The night continued with hugs and good wishes, and then, long after the sun set behind the mountain where Geronimo had done a vision quest more than a hundred years earlier, McNally led the retreatants into the darkness. Thorson strode beside her, carrying three plastic bags full of supplies. McNally's thin cotton robes fluttered in the gusts. Remarkably, at least in the video of her departure, she did not shiver.

The next morning, the couple woke up in their cottage under the sway of a mutual vow of silence. The Lama Dome's windows opened onto a majestic view of the retreat valley below. It was the highest building in the valley, and every retreatant could look up and see their teacher's home. If they'd had binoculars or a telescope, someone down below might have been able to make out Ian and Christie assuming acroyoga poses on their porch in the morning light. The architecture was meant to inspire the other residents of the valley and let them know they would never be alone on their spiritual journey.

Even though they couldn't talk, the retreat schedule at Diamond Mountain wasn't designed to be entirely asocial. It was divided into two-month blocks of intensive meditation, and then two-month blocks during which the retreatants could wander the compound and interact at silent meetings. No one was permitted to speak, but they could pass written notes to one another and post letters to the outside world. The retreatants had consecrated the boundaries of the retreat valley in a holy ritual and vowed not to cross its borders. In Tibetan, the ritual barriers were called a *tsam,* and in tantric logic, the borders were a sort of echo chamber that amplified their collective spiritual energy.

During the downtime between intensive periods, the retreatants took on clandestine projects. At night a group of them carved a snaking path to the summit of the mountain that overlooked the retreat, dubbed Tara Mountain, after the Tibetan goddess. The path worked its way over the east side of the retreat valley and through federal land. It stopped halfway up at an abandoned mine shaft that had been worked in the time of the Union army and overlooked the crumbled walls of historic Fort Bowie. The retreatants stashed pickaxes and ritual implements in the crevasse, along with a couple of wooden planks that could be used as a bed in a pinch. By day the path was within view of the ranger station, so they worked at night to ensure that the rangers wouldn't catch and arrest them for altering the landscape of a national park. At least one retreatant tweaked the rules of her own retreat and arranged to meet her lover in the cave in order to not bring him onto the official sanctified grounds.

When rangers nearby discovered the path, they were amazed by the amount of effort that had gone into it. They had the power to fine Diamond Mountain the $50,000 that it would cost to send maintenance crews up the mountain to erase the trail, but memories of the shoot-out at Miracle Valley still haunted relations between the government and fringe religious groups in Cochise County. For now, the Park Service was willing to let the retreatants meander up to the top of the mountain at night as long as most visitors to the park never learned of the trail's existence.

Soon, however, conflict seemed almost inevitable. In March 2011, three months after the beginning of the retreat, Christie and Ian descended from their house on the hill, Ian limping as they crossed the road that cuts across the retreat valley, holding a bloody cloth to his side. Together they knocked on the door of a nurse-practitioner who was on the retreat with them and asked for help. Blood oozed out around the cloth from three separate stab wounds.

No one offered an explanation for how the cuts got there, but they sank deeply into the skin between his ribs and across his shoulders and seemed serious enough to have threatened vital organs. The nurse turned Ian and Christie away, worried the damage was beyond her abilities—or, even worse, that she might be viewed as an accomplice to a crime. Afraid the wounds might result in a police report if they went to a hospital, the couple hobbled to their second choice: a dermatologist named Renee Miranda, who reluctantly tended to the slashes and stab wounds with precise stitches.

The wounds were supposed to be a secret, but rumors of domestic abuse circulated in the same hushed-whisper circles that had described sexual liaisons between Roach and his various students almost ten years before. The sense of unease permeated the upper retreat valley.

Then, one day, they looked up and saw black smoke on the horizon. As the year marched onward toward the summer, the sun had baked the water out of the dry ground, leaving the washes barren and scrubby juniper bushes desiccated and easy tinder. In June, a horseshoe-shaped wildfire scorched its way across the mountain valleys in what was just one of several fires that were sweeping across almost half a million acres of Arizona. The *New York Times* dispatched a reporter to see how the retreatants planned to deal with the blaze. The reporter met with Scott Vacek, who said he'd consider evacuation, but only as a last resort.

"They can see the smoke coming over the hill," said Scott Vacek, one of the caretakers on the property and also a practicing Buddhist. "It looks startlingly close. But we haven't told them that we may be coming in to

evacuate them. We didn't see any upside to that, because their meditations will immediately be over. They wouldn't be able to concentrate."

—*The New York Times,* June 17, 2011

The fire blackened the sky and reached the rim of the valley but didn't cross over the line of the *tsam*. There was a feeling that their efforts meditating and casting their will over nature had kept the fire at bay. But the close call could have also been a warning.

It wasn't until March 2012 when McNally had a chance to take the stage, just as she did in St. David a decade earlier, that anyone in the outside world could catch a glimpse of the inner workings of the three-year retreat.

For the event, cooks, volunteers, yogis, and meditators set up tents on the rocky ground in the lower valley and booked the few hotel rooms in the nearby cowboy town of Willcox. The three-day event was heavy on fund-raising sales pitches as the board of directors scrambled for money that would let them continue the retreat indefinitely. They offered free yoga classes in the central temple and guided meditations. At least one hundred cars overflowed into a hastily bulldozed parking lot, and at times there were so many people in the temple that they continued out the back door.

As before, a heavy curtain separated retreatants from the rest of the audience, and when any of them came to the stage, they wore a blindfold over their eyes and spoke with heavy, unused voices. It seemed that some were surprised by the sound of their own voice. Lectures by retreatants and caretakers lasted for three days. At the climax, McNally appeared from behind the curtain in her white robes, smiling beautifully from behind her yellow silk blindfold. Michael Roach had skipped the first two days of the event but made a special point to attend his ex-wife's talk. A live web feed connected McNally to her followers around the world.

At first, the talk seemed as though it would go unremembered except by a few zealous students—just another explanation of the mysterious clockwork of karmic seeds and her own burning desire to see emptiness directly. McNally recollected her personal tutelage under Roach and her years by his side, starting with the first retreat. "If your lama doesn't like something you are doing, he whacks you over the head," and on occasion, "Geshe Michael did that with me," she said. It was a starting point for unpacking the wounds that she'd left on Thorson's body.

For Christie and Ian, the retreat was an opportunity to understand violence at a deeply personal level. People in the audience nodded as they recollected Thorson's outbursts, and McNally noted that as they settled into the routine of daily meditations, an "aggressive energy" built up in their relationship. They prayed to Kali for help and realized that to master this energy, they would have to first build their feelings of aggression and violence rather than attempt to subdue the flames. So they began to play. McNally said she assumed the role of Kali and armed herself with a kitchen knife that she'd received as a wedding gift. She felt the deity's energy course through her body as she tried to visualize perfect aggression. She became the wrathful deity as the two of them assumed fighter poses and focused their minds somewhere between meditation and combat readiness.

We are sparring with each other like martial artists in silence and tension. I'm sort of hesitant to engage, and not sure of this particular playground. He hands me a knife, a big knife, and was daring me, "Go for it," you know. I came towards my partner with this knife because that's what I was supposed to do. He was supposed to stop me. He was supposed to grab my wrist, but for some strange reason he just let go and stopped fighting. Then the knife came down, and it actually cut into his flesh. I didn't notice at first. And he grabs me in some kind of embrace and the knife accidentally comes down again—accidentally, I don't know. He falls to the floor. Then she [Kali] leaves and the blood starts to come and I drop the knife.

"Oh, what have I done?"

I'm in my mind, when I came at my partner with a knife (it's a funny thing to say). I had one thought of my own in the back of my mind amidst all that energy; it was, "I must not harm him." I think that probably saved his life.

Then, afterwards I was like, "It was an accident!" But how can it be an accident when my hand was the one holding the knife? I looked at him and I asked, "What were you doing? Why didn't you stop me? Why didn't you stop me?" All the tension was gone and his eyes were totally clear and he looked up at me like he was really happy with me.

He said, "I trust you."

So we went down our hill to go look for somebody to sew up his body. It was a big gash. Afterwards when, when we got home, I took the knife, and . . . it was an object that could not any longer stay in our house. So I put it back in its little box and I wrapped it up and I put it in the outside closet, because I didn't want it anywhere near us. Every time I looked at it, it made me nauseous.

Reality had set in when the vision of herself as Kali faded. Her "holy love" was a wounded man and she had difficulty reconciling her role in the injury. Her hand held the weapon but, she maintained, the fault of the incident lay somewhere else. Perhaps the knife was the culprit.* That Ian let down his defenses at that crucial moment spoke either to a masochistic streak or to his willingness to tease the boundaries of death itself. Ian stayed hidden behind the curtain during her lecture, and no one had a chance to record his reaction.

Later, in a teaching titled "A Shift in the Matrix," she would write of the event, "My love was learning to deal with being in a relationship with someone who had a lot more power than him. At the beginning it was difficult and he broke down on occasions." She wrote that they invoked Kali and "when the accident happened, my Love said he felt like it was an answer to our prayers."

Sierra Shafer, a twentysomething devotee with red dreadlocks down to her waist who had recently graduated from Reed College, remembered a collective gasp from the listeners, but no one knew what to make of McNally's speech. Tantric lessons often contradicted

---

*In anthropology this sort of reasoning echoes a vein of fetishistic magic that credits inanimate objects with powers unto themselves. For instance, the saying "Hair of the dog that bit you," which is used nowadays to describe a way to cure a hangover, by consuming more alcohol the next day, originates from an ancient belief that the best cure to stave off an infection from a dog bite was to actually consume its hair.

common sense. Was this so different from the time that Roach asked McNally to stick her hand in a fire? They looked to Roach for guidance, but he kept silent immediately after her speech and left for his residence as quickly as possible.

Some people thought that perhaps this speech was a postmarital spat being played out in public lectures. Roach looked for answers in his meditations and looked to his angels for guidance. The next day, he held a public meeting that denounced McNally's violent liturgy. He asserted to the board his intention to take back control of the community from his charismatic ex-wife.*

The board filed a police report with the Cochise County Sheriff's Department and included an excerpt of McNally's speech. Jigme Palmo, a nun who, at least on paper, was charged with the care of the retreatants, worried what might become of Diamond Mountain if news leaked, or if there was another incident. "It was an impossible situation," said Palmo several months later. "We didn't know what was happening inside the retreat." Since they were barred from entering the *tsam*, there was no easy way to know what McNally was teaching the other thirty-eight people. The board consulted a lawyer and sent urgent written messages to McNally, asking for more information about possible domestic violence and her increasingly erratic decisions. News of the violence was leaking out to the broader community, and it was better to police their own flock than let outsiders do it for them.

They requested written statements from retreatants. McNally tried to shore up control of the meditators by banning all correspondence with the outside world. She ordered all mail deliveries to cease and instructed the retreatants even to refuse contact with their families. The board hung on the words of Michael Roach as spiritual director of Diamond Mountain. He denounced McNally, saying that she had drifted too far from the central teachings, and urged the board to unilaterally remove her from her position as retreat leader and expel her from the land.

---

*Board member Nicole Davis offered a different narrative of the events after the speech. "Geshe Michael Roach never asserted to the board that he needed to take back control. There was a lengthy board process following the speech and the board decided on a direction together after considering all options exhaustively."

They erased the online record of the speech and began to purge any online connection that McNally had to the group, just as they had with Michael Gordon of Bumble and Bumble. The goal was to remove any trace that McNally was ever involved with Diamond Mountain. Websites that once proudly displayed the monk and his wife lecturing side by side returned blank results.

Later, McNally told a reporter that "Geshe Michael told another group of people that I was the dangerous one. Dangerous for him, perhaps."

Scott Vacek and Rob Ruisinger, president of the board of directors, drove a pickup truck through the valley to deliver the message in person. Christie and Ian sat in the same room that, a year earlier, had been covered in Ian's blood. They worked as a team, planning for contingencies and frantically scratching out notes to each other. They heard the truck crunch its way over the gravel and peeked outside to see the board members approaching. Unaccustomed to unannounced visitors, McNally sensed what she later called an "evil intent." The couple ran to the bathroom and hid next to their cast-iron tub. The men knocked but, failing to receive an answer, tacked two letters to the door. McNally later paraphrased the notes' contents this way.

"The board has voted. You are no longer retreat leader here. You are no longer Spiritual Director of Diamond Mountain. You have an hour to leave Diamond Mountain property. If you do not leave within the hour, we will call the sheriff and have you forcibly removed. He is standing by."

Leaving a silent retreat can feel a little like resurfacing after a deep-sea dive; coming up to the surface too quickly can be jarring and psychologically devastating. Roach and the board knew that proper protocol dictated letting people leave a retreat in gradual stages, but they were more concerned with the potential political fallout than with any consequences that might befall Christie or Ian.

Though the outside world was marshaling against her, the silence inside the retreat valley still gave McNally some power. As far as anyone there cared, she was still leader inside the *tsam*. Together the couple traveled to the retreat yurts of her students and organized a letter-writing campaign to force the board to revise their order. Most students in the retreat had taken McNally as a lama in at least one of their initiations. To go against her would be to break one of their highest tantric vows. It didn't take long for them to show support.

With the people in the valley behind her, McNally and the board haggled like merchants in an Asian bazaar. The board relented and offered to cover her hotel costs, a rental car, a pair of prepaid cell phones, and provide $3,600 in cash—as long as she cleared off the land within five days. Maybe the couple could go back to the Bahamas and lead retreats there, or to meditation centers in Colorado or Kathmandu, where they would no doubt find an audience for their philosophy. Whatever her solution, she would have to give up her students at Diamond Mountain and hand them over to the spiritual responsibility of Michael Roach.

McNally needed help. She turned to a monk whom she had given the name Chandra and a former investment banker named Akasha, both of whom she thought would be loyal to her no matter what. The two had worked as caretakers at Diamond Mountain and could help manage arrangements for McNally and Thorson to reenter the world once they left the retreat. Chandra had tattoo sleeves covering what some people at Diamond Mountain claimed were the scars of a past heroin addiction. He'd been a chef at a Houston restaurant and didn't always pay back the money other students lent him. Akasha had been born in India and moved to New York, where he had attempted to design quantitative models that would predict the movements of the stock market. When that failed he looked to the desert to pursue a more contemplative life.

McNally instructed the two attendants to purchase supplies for an extended stay in the desert. She and Thorson would need camping gear and whatever else it would take to live a rustic existence. If Roach wouldn't let them finish the three-year commitment on Diamond Mountain land, they could still try to finish what they started somewhere nearby.

Technically, the consecrated lines of the *tsam* extended past the official property line of Diamond Mountain. The sacred loop included the places where Geronimo had once roamed across the top of Tara Mountain. The couple could live like the Indians and use the sacred energy of the earth to achieve enlightenment on their own. If they were successful, who would be able to question their commitment to the dharma or the righteousness of their actions?

Akasha drove to an upscale camping store in Tucson and bought several thousand dollars' worth of gear with his own money. Everything was lightweight and top of the line. He added a satellite locator beacon to their emergency supplies, a cell phone with a solar charger, and a water filter just in case either McNally or her husband got into trouble.

In her search for allies, McNally met with Michael Brannan, who had long been feeling uneasy with the teachings at Diamond Mountain. At the time, Brannan was in charge of stocking the Sub-Zero refrigerator with fresh vegetables while he pursued his own idiosyncratic meditations in a trailer back in Bowie. They sat down together and wrote notes back and forth on loose-leaf paper, creating an effective transcript of her thoughts at that moment.

Brannan now keeps the notes safe and folded like a holy relic. He is at once protective and wistful about McNally. It was plain that he is jealous of Ian Thorson's speedy ascendancy.

The two conversed in a hurried script. McNally wrote that she was determined to have a new start. The conditions in the retreat had made her feel like a prisoner and she would be happy to be out from under Roach's spell. She hadn't expected the forceful reaction of the board to her speech, but she was positive that her expulsion was just temporary and part of a broader plan. "Everything is perfect, you will see," she wrote, adding, "I have inherited my holy lama's [Geshe Michael] style of pushing people past their breaking point." She blamed her former husband for "stoking the fire" and making people fear her as a teacher.

More so than anything else, though, the note seethes with a palpable fear that the decision might put her in danger. "Now I will be in retreat alone with Ian with no one to run to—how is that 'protecting' me?" she asked. She called Ian "profoundly undisciplined and spoiled" but said that he was changing for the better in the retreat. She asked how, if people suspected the couple of being violent toward each other, being alone together in a cave without supervision would be any safer?

The letter ended with McNally asking Brannan to leave her alone so her attendants could meet privately and discuss the details of her next move. That night she and Thorson walked out into the desert with just a few supplies on their backs. The only two people who knew where they were headed took a vow to keep their destination secret.

Part 3

The Dark Night of the Soul

The Suicide Sutra

A Buddhist Parable

THE BUDDHA HADN'T *blazed the path to enlightenment so much as he'd blundered upon it. There was a difference between knowing the ultimate laws of the universe and being able to explain it to others. It turned out that he still had something to learn about being a teacher.*

It was a problem of pedagogy.

Since he'd achieved enlightenment, the Buddha had been busy teaching his philosophy to students in present-day Nepal and Bihar. As he saw it, one of the major stumbling blocks to enlightenment was that his students were so attached to their own bodies that they couldn't grasp the subtle truth about death and rebirth. The key to understanding karma, he thought, was to first show his students that their bodies were impermanent. If they could face the reality of their own deaths, then perhaps they would understand that even mortality is empty of any deeper meaning.

In those days not every corpse was buried or burned. When they died, paupers, criminals, and prostitutes rotted in putrid fields called charnel grounds on the outskirts of every town. They sat exposed to the elements and decayed in the open. Worms wiggled in the bloated eye sockets and pus oozed from their seven bodily orifices.

At a stopover at one monastery, the Buddha told his students to go to the charnel ground, not only to see the bodies, but also to see the cemetery as a second sort of monastery. He commanded his devotees to meditate in the muck of decay and visualize how their own bodies would one day rot in the morass.

Sure that they would grasp the new lesson, the Buddha went to meditate on his own in a nearby cave and asked not to be disturbed.

The monks did as they were told. They marched to the putrefied field and meditated on the corrupted flesh. But they did not arrive at the peaceful place that the Buddha had promised they would. Instead of liberation from the constraints of death, many monks began to feel that their own bodies were no different from the dead ones in front of them. If death was so certain, why not embrace it? Soon, the monks wanted nothing more than to shed their skin and enter their next life. Perhaps they would find enlightenment on the other side.

It was too much for one monk and he committed suicide by slitting his own throat. Another followed his example. Soon there was a full-blown epidemic. Thirty monks took their own lives every day. Those who were unable to do the deed themselves urged other monks to do it for them.

The congregation was caught in the grip of a grim reverie. The holy men elected a disciple named Migalandika to become their chief executioner. He used a knife to slit their throats. At first he killed only those who asked for release. However, as his desire to help other people achieve enlightenment grew, he traveled from monastery to monastery, killing monks as they meditated. They died in their chambers and in charnel grounds. The Buddhists welcomed him as an angel of death.

Several months later the Buddha returned from his solitude to find most of his flock decaying in the field around him. The few survivors shook with fear and disbelief. If this was the path to enlightenment, then what was the point? The Buddha's attendant Ananda begged his teacher to devise a new method for reaching Nirvana.

The story is recounted in the Vinaya—the same set of teachings that lists the vows every monk must take to receive ordination. The ancient account doesn't record the Buddha's reaction except to say that he assembled the remaining monks and told them to stop meditating on decaying corpses at once. He excommunicated Migalandika and admitted to the students who survived that there were other ways to grasp the impermanence of all things than facing their mortality so directly.

Instead of meditating on corpses, his devotees could grasp impermanence by silently concentrating on the rising and falling of their own breathing. The new technique became the Buddha's most powerful lesson and is still to this day the first form of meditation that teachers give to new students.

Buddhists remember the first lesson in the charnel grounds as one of the Buddha's few failures. He was a Bodhisattva and master of the laws of karma, but he was not infallible.

This little-known suicide sutra exists in only two Pali texts, and most practicing Buddhists may have never come across it. It remains a warning about the dangers that people face on the path to enlightenment.

13.

Spiritual Sickness

Siddhis *are beautiful, but they will bind us, because* siddhis *are the outcome of the mind. The mind* wants *something. It wants to achieve this or that. What for? To be proud of itself. It develops ego. It makes your "I" and "mine" bigger. Selfish desires are still there. If you are after* siddhis *like astral traveling, clairvoyance and clairaudience, I ask you why? You may say, "Oh, I thought I could help people." I say that is just an excuse. You want to show you can do something. To be proud of it.*
—Sri Swami Satchidananda
The Yoga Sutras of Patanjali

We are not human beings having a spiritual experience, but spiritual beings having a human experience.
—Pierre Teilhard de Chardin

AMY CAYTON WEARS her silver hair bobbed around her ears and crops her bangs to frame her face. She works out of a small second-floor office in a building designed to ape the woody lines of Craftsman architecture. She has a PhD in sociology, but her clients seek her out as a counselor for advice to clear up their marital problems. Patients fight addictions to alcohol, sex, love, and drugs.

If the case calls for it, she employs hypnosis and gently explores the subconscious. Sometimes she'll suggest that meditation might clear up the anxiety that seems to go hand in hand with the modern world. She credits Tibetan Buddhism with allowing her to embrace the simple truth that every living being deserves compassion. But the journey has not always been easy.

In 2002, she recited mantras on a three-week meditation retreat and something started to go wrong. At night she tossed and turned in her bed, and her mind kept spinning over the same anxious ideas. At breakfast she didn't feel like herself. By lunchtime she had trouble breathing. Then, as she hunched over a vegetarian meal, she began to gasp for air. A woman put her hand on Cayton's shoulder and gave her a diagnosis that she had never read in any of her psychological literature. The lady gave her a concerned look and said that Amy Cayton had *lung*: the meditator's disease.

"I was the sort of person who gave 110 percent to everything, and approached meditation the same way. Then *lung* set in and I was suddenly emotional over everything. I'd get angry over nothing, or just burst into tears. Western doctors couldn't diagnose the physical symptoms—shortness of breath, and loss of memory. And then there was exhaustion. The main thing was exhaustion." The smorgasbord of vague symptoms might match up with any number of anxiety disorders. She stopped eating. Stopped sleeping. Her descent put her into an existential drift that she described as "becoming more and more like herself." It was as if her own personality traits amplified themselves: Anger became rage; happiness, ecstasy; sadness, despair; and the more she tried to focus on the tool that she had relied on to fix things—meditation—the more her own focus thwarted her attempts. It was as if she were a living, breathing caricature of herself.

For centuries, if not millennia, Eastern medicine systems have held that the human body has two main components. There is the physical self of bones, blood, muscles, nerves, and hormones. And there is the subtle body that moves spiritual energy—*qi* in Chinese, or *prana* in Sanskrit—through riverlike pathways called *nadis*. Instead of a single heartlike pump, the subtle body has seven spinning vortexes called chakras that keep the energy moving through the system. Ultimately, energy moves through the body and out the crown of the head to a divine tether. When it's healthy, energy flows freely and *prana* moves smoothly through one chakra to another. But many things can go wrong along the way. When one chakra stops spinning, a channel can get blocked or the entire system can get out of alignment. Some advanced meditators try to consciously alter the energy body and condition themselves for particular types of enlightening experiences. If they are not careful, their manipulations can move energies in ways that can cause profound damage. *Lung* is one such condition.

Cayton approached Lama Zopa Rinpoche, the founder of the Foundation for the Preservation of the Mahayana Tradition (FPMT)—the same organization that ran the Root Institute in Bodh Gaya and introduced both Ian Thorson and Christie McNally to Tibetan Buddhism. Based on Cayton's symptoms, he suggested an aggressive regimen of Tibetan medicine. He instructed her to eat heavier foods and stop meditating for a while. It took time, but eventually her symptoms subsided.

When she recovered fully, Lama Zopa asked her to write a book about her experience and warn other Westerners about the potential dangers of *lung*, which he said in some cases might be devastating. The Tibetan word *lung* translates literally to "wind" and refers to the chaotic movements of wind energy through the subtle body. Her first project for the book was to reach out to FPMT LISTSERVs and web boards to ask people to record their own encounters with *lung*. The replies flooded in.

For some, the onset was a slow creeping like Cayton had felt. For others, it was as if they had been struck by an electric charge. A few of the most serious cases ended up in the wards of psychiatric hospitals, unable to differentiate the visions in their heads from the outside world. *Lung* doesn't present itself as a single codified disease but has a range of symptoms. Yet one thing is certain: It's a progressive condition that gets worse the longer it goes untreated. "In this way," she says, "*lung* is like any other mental ailment."

The FPMT published Cayton's book in 2007 under the title *Balanced Mind, Balanced Body: Anecdotes and Advice from Tibetan Buddhist Practitioners on Wind Disease*. The hundred-page booklet includes commentaries from monks who recount their eagerness to teach

Western students when they first arrived from Asia. Its pages illustrate the clash of cultures that played out on meditation cushions across the country when the FPMT was in its earliest days. In the sixties, seventies, and eighties, when teachers from Tibet first started arriving on Western shores, they were initially impressed by the brightness of their students, and by the material wealth and infrastructure of the countries. They were confident that their new students would excel at spiritual practice.

But things did not go as expected. Even relatively simple practices went awry when Western students tried to grapple with esoteric ideas. A few star pupils reported to their teachers that sitting for long periods of time caused them to feel overwhelmed with angst. Students shook. They couldn't sleep. It was only after seeing dozens of them have the same experience that the teachers realized something was wrong with their approach to meditation. Westerners, it turned out, could be too driven and too focused on attaining a final spiritual state. They took to meditation as if it were a job with a goal at the end. One of the commentaries in Cayton's book puts it succinctly: "People who only meditate for stress reduction or who aren't interested in attaining enlightenment probably don't often get *lung*. We get *lung* because we are trying to do something, to attain something, instead of relaxing and letting it happen naturally."

Most practitioners who responded to Cayton's request were already on the road to recovery. They'd seen their way through the darkest times and offered advice to other people in similar spots. Their solutions were as idiosyncratic as the symptoms. Some suggested taking a break from meditation and focusing more on yoga. Many offered dietary changes. They tried acupuncture, or prayers to different gods and goddesses. They recommended sex, or brandy. Or abstinence. One woman said she kicked *lung* only after she got pregnant. The one common thread was to break the routine. The one thing that everyone could agree on was that once *lung* had set in, more meditation would only make it worse.

Even though the evidence mounted in her in-box, Cayton is cautious not to blame meditation itself for the epidemic when I ask her about it. "The techniques can exacerbate an existing problem if the student isn't careful. This is why it's critically important that someone has a qualified teacher guiding them along and corrects a problem before it gets out of control."

Lung is just one of a series of maladies known to waylay people on the road to spiritual perfection. Another that some yoga practitioners describe is the sudden play of ecstasy and rage that happens when they start to experience new energies in their bodies, which they call the kundalini syndrome.

In 1975 a yogi named Gopi Krishna helped popularize the concept of kundalini to the world in his bestselling book *The Awakening of Kundalini*. According to age-old yogic texts, kundalini energy lies dormant near the base of the spine, in a place that corresponds to the bottommost chakra. It is a feminine libidinal force that, in its unawakened state, sits in several coils inside the anatomy of the subtle body. The energy is dormant in most people, but when it wakes up, the energy gushes up the spine like a snake and spills out the crown of the head, radically shifting a person's perspectives as it does. People who have had their kundalini awoken through meditation, yoga, traumatic experiences, or a guru's blessing often list it as one of the most profound and beautiful moments of their life.

Krishna wrote that kundalini energy isn't always positive. "The power, when aroused in a body not attuned to it with the help of various disciplines or not genetically mature for it, can lead to awful mental states, to almost every form of mental disorder, from hardly noticeable aberrations to the most horrible forms of insanity, to neurotic and paranoid states, to megalomania and, by causing tormenting pressure on reproductive organs, to an all-consuming thirst that is never assuaged." Other writers describe suddenly awakened people spontaneously assuming deep yoga poses, or obsessively performing ritual hand gestures called mudras.

Donald Lopez, the author and professor to whom Ian Thorson's parents turned for advice on the authenticity of Roach's teachings, has written that in the West the view of meditation is far too one-sided: "Where is the insistence that meditation is not intended to induce relaxation but rather a vital transformation of one's vision of reality?" he wrote in *Buddhism and Science: A Guide for the Perplexed*. As tools, the practices of kundalini yoga and intensive meditation are not necessarily aimed at making someone a more adaptable person in all social environments; rather, they can bring about drastic and sometimes unwieldy changes. Meditation and yoga might be better thought of as powerful, or transformative, rather than a set of practices that can only put someone on an upward trajectory.

Scientists have tried to understand what happens during meditation and yoga since at least 1970. In that year, Robert Keith Wallace, a young doctor at UCLA medical school, gathered together a group of transcendental meditators and hooked them up to monitoring devices that checked their oxygen levels, heart rates, skin resistance, and EEG results. The machines reported back almost immediate improvements, including better cardiovascular efficiency and changes in brain wave frequencies. While these results seem almost commonsense now, they were revolutionary at the time. Wallace took his study out for peer review and published the results in the journal *Science*. It was the first accredited research on meditation in a real journal. In the next two years, the study appeared on the covers of *Time* and *Scientific American* and effectively opened the floodgates of scientific inquiry into meditative states. Over the next forty years, hundreds of other studies followed suit.

Wallace's credentials include degrees from Harvard and some of the most prestigious medical centers in the country. What wasn't initially clear about his affiliations was that, in addition to being a careful researcher, Wallace was the founding president of the Maharishi University of Management in Iowa—the world headquarters of Transcendental Meditation.*

---

*Wallace and I are both descendants of the famous-in-his-time Massachusetts surgeon Philemon Truesdale, and technically, I believe, we are second cousins even though he hails from an older generation and I refer to him as an uncle. From time to time we have shared Thanksgiving dinners and engaged in lively conversations about heart disease, meditation, and potential links between psychosis and spiritual striving. Both black sheep of the family in our own ways, Wallace might be the reason I took an interest in meditation at a young age.

Wallace's first wife—let's call her Edna Wallace—was a magazine cover model and media "it" girl for a brief moment in the 1970s. After a child or two, they eventually split apart, but both con-

Transcendental Meditation is unusual in terms of Indian meditation systems because it unabashedly attempts to cultivate the power of levitation. At the center in Iowa, and on satellite campuses around the world, transcendentalists sit cross-legged and hop into the air while psychically attempting to make their bodies ethereal. So far, no transcendental meditator has been documented achieving the feat. In 1985, a group of former transcendental meditators banded together to sue Maharishi University for what amounted to false advertising. They had spent years and tens of thousands of dollars on course fees without ever achieving the superpowers they had been promised. Most of the people who filed suit eventually settled out of court, including the two exit counselors whom Ian's parents had hired to convince their son to leave Roach's sway.

As a category, research on meditation almost always shares a certain selection bias. Positive results get attributed to the meditation practices while negative ones are reduced to the status of preexisting conditions. Indeed, almost all researchers who focus on meditation are themselves avid meditators or yogis. In many cases spiritual institutions actually foot the bill for the studies in the first place.

Of course, Western medicine also has a reputation for selection bias against spiritual explanations. Mainstream scientists scoff at the thought that an undetectable parallel body could explain medical conditions. No conclusive scientific evidence charts the existence of energy pathways, and most empiricists would argue that much of what is attributed to the subtle body can be just as easily explained through

---

tinued to be active transcendental meditators. According to a newsletter written by ex-TM members who filed suit against Transcendental Meditation, Edna was attempting to master the feat of levitation and grew frustrated by her lack of progress. On February 6, 1984, she decided that another woman in her meditation group had been sapping her energy and preventing her from lifting off the meditation mat.

Once she had made up her mind to the cause, Edna left the center and bought a revolver, and at their next session together, Edna shot her nemesis while they meditated. Thankfully, the woman survived. Recently, when I spoke to my uncle, he denied the way the incident was described in the court case. She wasn't on Maharishi International University property, he said, and noted correctly that she had not been prosecuted; rather, she was treated for a mental condition.

Whether or not my ex-aunt was driven mad by Transcendental Meditation is a subject of speculation. Some people in my family say she was always a little strange. I mention the story to point out that much of the science done on meditation originates from sources who are already sold on the benefits of the practices. Negative results are often swept under the mat as incidental.

psychology or neuroscience. This may be true. However, at the moment, even the most cutting-edge tools of the neuroscientist—a variety of brain scans, questionnaires, EEGs, MRI scans, and CT scans—don't have the ability to show the connection between the mind and the body. There is no way to record a thought and read it out on a computer screen, or to identify the physical location of an emotion. We can only assume that somehow atoms and molecules add up to consciousness. This missing link between body and mind is a pernicious problem in modern medicine and neuroscience and leaves the door open to a variety of interesting, novel, and occasionally preposterous explanations.

Anyone who has tried Ayurveda, Reiki, or acupuncture—or, some would argue, even benefited from the placebo effect—has dipped a toe in the world of energy medicine. In the wake of record numbers of cases of post-traumatic stress disorder among returning veterans, even the military began prescribing acupuncture to treat the psychologically wounded vets. Many insurance companies will cover the cost of Reiki treatments or visits to the chiropractor. That these forms of medicine work, at least some of the time, is beyond doubt.

Still, one of their selling points is that alternative and energy medicine don't generally have any negative side effects other than that sometimes people will turn to alternative medicine when standard medicine for a particular ailment might be proven to save lives. Very few people enter into spiritual practices with awareness of the potential pitfalls. And for patients who lack intimate knowledge of the causes and treatments, things can go awry extremely quickly.

Ignoring the problem of potential bias, today a casual search for the word *meditation* on PubMed, a government-run medical website, shows almost 2,955 peer-reviewed scientific papers on meditation. A further 2,500 include the term *yoga*. Results indicate that the practices can be a panacea for any number of maladies far beyond simply cardiology. A 2014 study in the *Journal of the American Medical Association* found that out of 18,000 citations in medical literature, only 47 studies had a control group and were good enough to stand up to scientific scrutiny. The findings say a lot about how much we hope meditation might give us versus how much we can actually prove.

Nonetheless, the scientific interest only seems to grow. Researchers have hooked monks up to diagnostic equipment to show increases in empathy and neuroplasticity (the ability of the brain to adapt to new conditions). Another study shows that prisoners are better able to adapt to their restrictive environment if they meditate. Other people seem to be able to mentally control their blood pressure. Meditation might even ward off dementia in old age.

Cutting-edge research in the field of epigenetics notes that meditation might actually be able to change someone's genetic profile. One study supported by Deepak Chopra shows that telomeres, the spindly ends of DNA that unravel slowly and irreparably with age, can be wound back up again with daily mental practice. If the findings hold up—Chopra, as a well-known meditation guru, has a vested interest in the results—it might mean that people could vastly extend the length of their lives.

It's much more difficult to find reliable studies that even define what negative reactions might look like. In 1999, an Australian psychological journal proposed an update to the *Diagnostics and Statistics Manual of Mental Disorders* IV (DSM-IV) with a condition known as Qigong-induced psychosis to describe meditators in this Chinese tradition who suddenly and seriously turn unstable. A 1984 study, by Stanford University psychologist Leon Otis, of 574 subjects involved in Transcendental Meditation showed that 70 percent of longtime meditators displayed signs of mental disorders. Neuroscientists have discovered that over the long term, meditating can cause changes in the composition of brain matter, and even short stints can create significant physical alterations in one's neurological makeup. Usually this is framed in terms of positive results.

Whatever changes occur during short, daily meditations are only amplified on silent retreats. Although comprehensive clinical studies on the potential adverse side effects of such retreats are just getting under way (one led by Willoughby Britton, a neuroscientist at Brown

University, is, at the time of this writing, in its second year), it is clear that some people find the isolation and mental introspection too intense. Some lose touch with reality or fall into psychotic states.

Since we don't really know what happens at a synaptic level—diagnostic machines that do exist are far too crude to analyze the brain in the sort of detail that could differentiate physical processes from more ephemeral ones—the best way we can understand the negative fallout of meditative experiences is through the words of meditators themselves.

Meredith Sagan is an unusual type of psychiatrist specializing in the treatment of spiritual anxiety disorders from an office in the hippie haven of Santa Monica, California. She started her spiritual journey back in 1992 at an ashram in Pune, India, that draws tens of thousands of Westerners every year. From there she dabbled in various spiritual movements, taking classes in Zen, communing with South American shamans, and learning to channel Vajrayogini with a Tibetan lama. Every move to a new esoteric tradition taught her a different set of skills and delivered transcendent experiences that conditioned her to grasp at a spirit world just beyond her fingertips.

Her journey spanned twenty years, and she reports that she was always looking for the next touch of the divine. Adept at retreats, she traveled to Chiang Mai, Thailand, where she had learned of a group of people called breatharians, who believe—and teach—that it is possible to become so attuned to the movement of energy throughout the world that they can live on air alone. Breatharians forgo food and supposedly sustain themselves on the nectar of the world, literally sucking *prana* from the sky.

Sagan decided that she'd give it a try, and so, with a handful of other ascetics, she plunged into total darkness. Though it was in a meditation compound, the room was made to feel like the interior of a cave. It was cold, damp, and pitch-black. The total sensory deprivation let her ignore her body so she could focus entirely on her own inner light.

After a few days, all she could feel was the crushing pain of intense hunger. Her body craved food and gnawed at her from the inside. In time, however, even those sensations ceased to be important. The pain was there, but it backed off. She felt herself move to higher realms until she experienced the release from her body as bliss. She felt euphoric.

Sagan felt herself drifting away up and out of the cave itself. She describes the feeling as being immersed in "multidimensional reality of emptiness." There were whole days of euphoria as she contemplated the bliss of the universe. Then her body began to call her back. The pangs of hunger returned and insisted that she come to the real world or pay a real-world price.

Torn between pain and bliss, Sagan knew she had a choice. Her mind was not her body, but they were still connected. She felt that she could cut the tether and continue to experience bliss. Her body would die, but her mind would continue onward. Or she could come back and reassert ownership of her physical self. It was hard to decide, but later that day she limped out of the darkness.

Breatharianism wreaked havoc on her digestive system. In her body's struggle to stay alive, her metabolic system dissolved her muscles and digested her stomach lining. The damage was real and it took months before she could eat properly again.

Yet, through the pain of recovery, Sagan found something she hadn't realized she was seeking. In the years of her spiritual wanderlust, her relationships with her family and friends had fallen into tatters: all sacrificed for internal transcendence. "I was a great yogini, knew how to meditate and to access states of awareness and bliss, but the one thing I didn't know how to do was have a healthy relationship," she recalls. Sensing ultimate reality made her wonder if it mattered whether or not the world was a delusion. "What good is consciousness if you can't interface with the masses?" she asks today.

So after twenty years of spiritual experimentation, Sagan returned to the world to finish her PhD and begin counseling people who were locked in their own spiritual conundrums. In the psychological literature, she found a diagnosis called spiritual bypassing, which enabled her to analyze the importance of her epiphanies.

The field of psychology doesn't have anything to say about the ultimate truth of any one experience or event, but it can say a lot about how one person's actions affect a group. The pursuit of spiritual goals can be a useful excuse to avoid dealing with painful feelings, unresolved trauma, and limited professional development. But prioritizing transcendence over relationships becomes a way to be self-centered while appearing to be concerned for the benefit of other people. So psychologists like Sagan apply a simple test to spiritual statements: Do the beliefs and practices take the person closer to a functional and helpful existence, or away from one?

For practitioners who hyperfocus on their inner life, the external world can fall away. They might limit their external stimuli so that all they see is their mind. Another way to radically transform the inner self is to travel to a completely foreign environment to kick-start a profound experience. As with the hajj or a Christian pilgrimage, a journey can be a spiritual experience in itself.

For people attuned to spiritual experiences, being in a landscape enriched by religious symbols can be a powerful boon to their practice. In the age of cheap international travel, it's increasingly easy for anyone to travel across the world to the spots where the Buddha or Krishna once walked. Getting to India and Tibet no longer requires dangerous treks across mountains or endless months on a boat.

In 2010, nearly 5.8 million people, including about 930,000 Americans, traveled to India. Roughly a quarter of all tourists at least dabble in India's spiritual industries—attending a meditation seminar or taking a religious pilgrimage of one sort or another. A tourist has thousands of options to choose from: Pilates-inspired yoga at five-star hotels, intensive retreats that combine the Hindu health system of Ayurveda with complex theological teachings. A visitor can marvel at ancient temple architecture or walk in the footsteps of the Buddha. Many programs cater specifically to Westerners. Some, like the Osho Ashram in Pune, won't even let Indian passport holders enter the grounds. In some ways, India is a sort of spiritual playground, with low costs and opportunity for all sorts of religiously inspired programs. Offerings accommodate just about any budget: A backpacker can spend a dollar a night to live in communal guesthouses at some Hindu and Sikh temples—called *dharamshalas*—or a well-heeled traveler can fork over thousands a night for an eco-friendly spa.

Some people are drawn by accounts of the powers of dedicated practitioners: yogis who can levitate, survive for months while entombed underground, or melt giant swaths of snow with their body heat. There are more than a few gurus who claim that they will unlock similar powers for any person who bows at their feet.

While not everyone heads to Asia with those goals in mind, the quest to become superhuman—along with culture shock, emotional isolation, illicit drugs, and the physical toll of hard-core meditation—can cause seekers to lose their bearings. Traveling abroad can be as destabilizing as journeying inside a tantric painting. Seemingly sane people get out of bed one day claiming they've discovered the lost continent of Lemuria, or that the end of the world is nigh, or that they've awakened their third eye. Most recover, but some become permanently delusional. A few vanish or even turn up dead.

Jonathan Spollen, a twenty-eight-year-old Irishman with long brown hair and a delicate brogue, was at a crossroads in his life. He'd embarked on a career as an overseas journalist, working first as a reporter at the *Daily Star Egypt* in Cairo and then as a foreign editor at *The National* in Abu Dhabi. Eventually, he took a job as a copy editor for the *International Herald Tribune* in Hong Kong. As he closed in on thirty, Spollen wondered if he liked where his life was going. In October 2011, following a split with his girlfriend, he bought some trekking gear, sent his laptop home to Dublin, and booked a flight to Kathmandu, Nepal. From there, he made his way to India. He had visited before, spending time with an octogenarian yogi named Prahlad Jani—who claimed his mastery of the ancient arts had allowed him to live without food for seventy years—and had come away entranced with the country.

This time, Spollen roamed the subcontinent for several months, following the Ganga River, first at Varanasi, India's oldest inhabited settlement. In early February 2012, Spollen called his mother, Lynda, to tell her he planned to spend two or three weeks hiking in the Himalayas near the pilgrimage site of Rishikesh, the yogaphilic city just down the river where the Beatles had visited Maharishi Mahesh Yogi in the 1960s. She reportedly asked him not to go alone, but he told her that was the whole point. "It's a spiritual thing," he explained.

He was never heard from again.

A little over three weeks after that conversation, his parents were worried enough to post to IndiaMike.com, a forum for Western travelers to the subcontinent. Their message contained a picture of Spollen, the details of his last known sighting, and a plea: "Please, all of you, keep in regular contact with your families. Even if they don't say it, they care for you and worry about you!" A few days later, Spollen's father, David, flew to Rishikesh to organize a search party. In mid-March, local authorities found Spollen's passport, rucksack, bedroll, and cash beside a waterfall near the village of Patna, only a few miles outside Rishikesh. From there, however, the trail went cold. Members of the IndiaMike community circulated missing-person posters that travelers hung along the Banana Pancake Trail, a network of backpacker routes that stretches from Goa to Hanoi. But there were no new leads.

The thread on the Spollens' initial post grew to more than 1,700 responses in a matter of months. Some commenters believed that he had died while others speculated that he chose to renounce his previous life and is still living in the mountains somewhere, alone or with some cloistered sect. Many presumed that whatever happened to him, his "spiritual thing" was responsible.

They'd seen it before: Some remembered Ryan Chambers, a twenty-one-year-old Australian spiritual seeker who visited ashrams before vanishing from Rishikesh in 2005, leaving his passport, wallet, and cell phone behind in his hotel room, along with a note that read, "If I'm gone, don't worry. I'm not dead, I'm freeing minds. But first I have to free my own."

Other pilgrims had been taken in by false gurus who lured them with sham spirituality, who drained their bank accounts and sometimes even imprisoned them against their will. In March, just weeks after Spollen's disappearance, Nepalese police freed a thirty-five-year-old Slovakian woman who reportedly had been held captive for two months by the followers of a man claiming to be the reincarnated Buddha. Neeru Garg, the district police chief of the nearby city of Dehradun, says of his ongoing investigation into Spollen's disappearance, "We are concentrating on the ashrams and holy men in the area."

Stories like Spollen's feel like Eastern versions of *Into the Wild*, the 1996 book about Chris McCandless, a young adventurer who died after trying to live off the land in Alaska. The tales of willful idealists whose romantic notions of remote lands lead them to embark on quixotic journeys all too frequently end in tragedy. In April 2010, Spollen wrote a travel story for *The National*, about spending time with a peasant family in Kashmir, that supports that interpretation: "The simplest things became fascinating," he wrote. "I found myself becoming enthralled in their lives. And strangely, I felt part of it all." Being in a foreign land seemed to factor into the spiritual appeal for Spollen. "He did have a strong interest in spirituality," a college friend remarked on IndiaMike. "It doesn't explain . . . why he's been incommunicado, but it could be an indication that people are searching along the right lines."

His father told an Irish newspaper in late April 2012 that visiting India was an eye-opening experience. "I have, at times, thought I was looking at somebody completely different to the son that I knew," he said. "To suddenly discover that there may be a whole spiritual aspect to his life that we hadn't really touched on is astonishing." Spollen never surfaced to describe the role that devotion played in his disappearance. But he fits the profile of the fervent young enthusiast of yoga, meditation, and Eastern thought who becomes lost—or worse—on a journey of spiritual self-discovery.

An unbroken lineage of erstwhile Westerners who have found wonder and inner fulfillment by heading east goes back at least to Marco Polo. Whether it was Jonathan Spollen, Emily O'Conner, Amy Cayton, Ian Thorson, Christie McNally, Michael Roach, Theos Bernard, or Madame Blavatsky, it wasn't enough to simply grapple with foreign spiritual ideas on their own, but actually being *in* India seems to have the power to create a new sense of self.

When the trip sparks a radical transformation, the psychosis even has a name: India syndrome. In 2000, the French psychiatrist Régis Airault wrote the definitive book on the phenomenon, *Fous de l'Inde*, which means "crazy about India." It relates his experiences as the staff psychiatrist for the French consulate in Mumbai, where he treated scores of his countrymen whose spiritual journeys took tragic turns. "There is a cultural fantasy at play," he explains. "[India syndrome] hits people from developed Western countries who are looking for a cultural space that is pure and exotic, where real values have been preserved. It's as if we're trying to go back in time."

Unfamiliar environments have long been known to bring on episodes of short-term delirium. In 1817, the French writer Stendhal described being physically overcome by the experience of viewing Florentine art; a century and a half later, the psychiatrist Graziella Magherini coined the term Stendhal syndrome (also called Florence syndrome) after treating patients who'd become dizzy and confused, even hallucinating or fainting, while visiting the Italian city, supposedly overcome by its beauty.

India syndrome is not an officially recognized disease, but many doctors are convinced it's real. Kalyan Sachdev, the medical director of Privat Hospital in New Delhi, says that his facility admits about a hundred delusional Westerners a year, many of whom had been practicing yoga around the clock. "There's the physical side of yoga and the psychic side, and sometimes people get it all out of order," he says. "Peaceful people can get aggressive even if they haven't taken any drugs." His treatment tends to be simple: Send them home as soon as possible. "People come to us with acute psychotic symptoms," he says. "But you put them on the plane and they are completely all right." Sunil Mittal, the head of the psychiatric unit at Cosmos Institute of Mental Health & Behavioral Sciences in New Delhi, reported that he had to send police to retrieve a California woman who'd overstayed her visa and refused to leave an ashram outside Rishikesh. There, Mittal says, she danced erotically in the courtyard each night for the yogis and was often observed in a "trancelike state." His prescription for her was also a return flight home where, when surrounded by a familiar environment, she recovered.

Often, however, more than just a plane ticket is required. Airault, who practices in Paris, recently treated a well-traveled, seemingly stable French optometrist in his thirties who'd begun having feelings of persecution after visiting the holy city of Pushkar—according to him, it began after he drank a bhang lassi, a hashish-infused yogurt shake that is part of many ecstatic religious rituals in India. From there he fled to the countryside, then to Mumbai, where he was found babbling about how the Church of Scientology was telling him to cut himself off from society. Back home in Paris, he was twice institutionalized and spent four years refusing to leave his house. "He was completely crazy, in a state of delirium, a psychosis that was set off by his trip to India," Airault said, adding that, through consultations, the man's condition eventually improved enough that he could hold down a job at a clothing store. The psychiatrist brushed off the suggestion that the patient might have developed the same problems even if he'd never left France. "It's important to understand that sometimes we go crazy in India because it's a culture too different from our own," he says. "It doesn't mean that we're mentally ill."

Jonathan Spollen's father returned home after several weeks in Rishikesh, but even several years later he and his wife kept up the search, maintaining a website and a Twitter feed (@FindSpollen) dedicated to locating their son. The frequency of posts on the India-Mike thread slowed over time, but in June 2010, after Spollen vanished, one commenter expressed his conviction that Spollen remained "holed up somewhere in the Himalayas with some *sadhus* and saints in search of spiritual salvation" and would return to his family once he'd found what he was looking for. All that's left of Spollen are stories he'd written online and the missing-person posters tacked up around Rishikesh. They bore two images of the young Irishman.

One, labeled 1 YEAR AGO, was of him smiling, fresh-faced and goateed, dressed in a shirt and jacket. The other, labeled 3 MONTHS AGO, showed the same man looking weary and gaunt, his features set, his expressionless eyes locked on the path ahead.

Inevitably when someone vanishes on a pilgrimage in a foreign land, or reacts erratically after an intensive yoga or meditation routine, there are two basic explanations: It could be that certain individuals are predisposed to mental instability; or was it the technique that made them mad? Genetic precursors for schizophrenia often begin to manifest in the late teens and early twenties, and intensive introspection, culture shock, or mental readjustments could be the final thing that pushes someone over the edge. Life is a preexisting condition, and without exhaustive evidence it's impossible to make a definitive statement. It could be that people who travel to India are already a self-selected minority. Perhaps, to some degree, any search for life's hidden meanings risks breaking with the status quo, and is one step closer to breaking with an otherwise meaningless existence.

One thing is indisputable: While a person can go on their own spiritual quest, the world continues without them. Meredith Sagan sat in a dark cave, eating only *prana,* and realized that life was a choice. She could stay in a state of bliss, a place where the broader community no longer mattered, or return to society and leave her transcendent experiences—no matter how real—behind her. Sagan chose life. Not everyone does.

Death on a Mountainside

*Just before we left to our retreat place in the sky, my Love and I sat on
the side of a craggy hill, tucked away in our sleeping bag, gazing out
over the retreat valley and wondering what will happen.*
—Christie McNally, "A Shift in the Matrix," April 19, 2012

LONG BEFORE THE Union army subdued Geronimo and ended the
last of the Indian Wars, before Spanish conquistadores crossed the
desert on horseback, before even the Apache staked their claim on
this parched landscape, an ancestor of the Pueblo Indians stashed a
large clay pot full of seeds inside a lonely mountain cave in what is
now Southeast Arizona. The pot was never recovered, so it sat there
absorbing the relentless summer rays and enduring at least a thousand winters, until one day it cracked at the bottom and spilled its
contents. If they hadn't already decomposed inside, the seeds would
have been a welcome meal for birds and rodents. A few might have
escaped their notice to sprout roots, only to be outcompeted by the
bristly cacti, yucca, agave, and sagebrush that are better adapted to
the loose gravel hillside. Out of the thousands of seeds in the pot,
perhaps one or two survived to maturity. If asked to explain why
some seeds perished while others flourished, Ian Thorson might have
replied that their individual fates were not dealt out at random. Like
all things, the seeds succeeded and failed according to their karma.
Just as karma would dictate Ian's fate here in the arms of his wife,
Lama Christie McNally.

When they came across it, they felt that the artifact connected their own expulsion from the retreat valley below to the long and violent history of the Apache forced from their land at gunpoint. It took several weeks for Ian to select just the right spot to finish the remaining two years of their silent retreat, and the pot was a sign.

They moved at night so no one would see them. They constantly scanned the valley floor for searchlights just in case their cover was blown. Only two people knew that they were still in the area. Weeks earlier, McNally sent a letter to the board of directors with a false plan. She wrote to them that she and Ian would leave the valley by car and stay at a hotel while she got her bearings. Her two attendants were key to pulling off the ruse.

Akasha and Chandra both wore maroon robes and they'd vowed that they would help McNally cover her tracks even while Chandra kept on with his normal duties in the kitchens and administrative buildings just outside the inner valley. Akasha had flown to Arizona from New York at McNally's request and awaited her instructions in a nearby hotel room. Akasha blacked out the address on the hotel receipt and submitted the document to the board for reimbursement.

It had taken McNally almost eight years and more than a million dollars to make the valley fit for habitation. She was proud of her achievement and in the first days of the retreat, she took a vow to stay within the sacred boundaries of the *tsam*. Yet, finishing the retreat in the wilderness was going to be a test of her faith. Chandra promised that he would deliver supplies when he could, but the mobile phone he gave her had spotty coverage at best. Circumscribed by secrecy, he'd have to sneak out to the couple with no one noticing and find their small campsite by starlight.

In the first year, the group of thirty-eight retreatants had worked tirelessly in secret to carve the dirt path past an abandoned mine shaft and eventually all the way up to the summit of Tara Mountain, almost eight thousand feet above sea level. It snaked along the border of Diamond Mountain property and public land operated by the Bureau of Land Management. At the top the Buddhists strung long ropes of brightly colored prayer flags, each stamped with Tibetan mantras meant to aid the progression of all sentient beings toward enlightenment. Somehow Christie and Ian sledged several Rubbermaid containers of basmati rice, cooking pots, ritual drums, and sleeping bags up the trail.

For the first few nights, the two holed up in their tent just out of sight of Fort Bowie. That time of year the weather was unreliable and few visitors to the old fort went off the main trails to explore the wilderness. There was more than enough space for them to keep hidden if no one came looking for them. But the tent was temporary protection from the elements at best. The desert gets cold at night and sometimes the wind can bear down on the thin fabric so heavily that it can make the flimsy structure collapse. Barring that, the noise from the tent fly whipping on the roof was enough to keep the inhabitants up all night.

Christie wasn't used to the rugged conditions. Ian, however, happily tromped around the jagged ridges of Tibet and was an inveterate explorer of the Chiricahua range. During the task of searching out a more permanent shelter, Ian became more than equal to his wife. Where he had relied on her spiritual guidance, this challenge was his to deliver hard results. One option he could have chosen was the small abandoned mine shaft. It extended thirty feet into the bedrock, and retreatants had used it to store their tools. Christie and Ian may have spent a few nights there, but they knew that someone would eventually come across them. They needed someplace secret.

So Ian climbed over boulders and across tan-colored rocks, looking for something better. Relics from Apache warriors and soldiers of the past turned up in the crevasses. Rifle shells, broken bottles, and metal parts all survived well in the dry air. One morning, Ian left Christie behind and descended the summit. He covered loose ground and picked his way around the spearlike fronds of agave and past the ominous rattling of poisonous snakes. There, in a depression between two soft ridgelines, he found what might have been the perfect spot.

The cave was a stony gash on the face of the mountain. It had a packed dirt floor left over from ancient occupants. The cracked pot had gone undisturbed since before Europeans had set foot in Arizona. The cave, in this sense, was a blessing. The black soot scars of ancient cooking fires on the wall connected them to the times of Geronimo. Of all the other caves nearby, the couple knew this one was special.

"We were sure that the one we were sleeping in must have belonged to the chief, and the rest of the tribe were in slightly less luxurious abodes. In any case, it was quite clear that no one had been there since the time of the Apaches," McNally wrote in a letter to *Rolling Stone*. Her assumption was off by at least five hundred years. An archaeologist from the Arizona State Museum who examined the pot noted that its flat gray slip suggested an even more ancient origin. Most likely it belonged to the Hohokam—Pueblo ancestors whom the Apache drove from the valley.

The cave was just tall enough for Thorson to extend his full six-foot, one-inch frame. There was room for them to drag a futon inside and create a habitable, if cramped, living space. They found a second small cleft in the rock, hidden behind a scraggy live oak about fifty feet below. They used it to store extra supplies. All told, they believed it was a suitable spot for a plan that was as elegant as it was dangerous: They would occupy the cave until they achieved enlightenment.

Over the course of the next two months rain, snow, and relentless 110-degree sun battered their secluded spot. Yet the weather didn't disturb their daily meditation routine. Christie doffed her trademark white robes and acceded to water-repellant hiking shorts and T-shirts. Water was scarce in the mountains, but Ian came up with an ingenious solution. He draped a tarp across a cleft above the cave's mouth so that dew and rain could collect on the fabric and filter down into a plastic jug. The water was earthy and brown but seemed palatable. For them the runoff and snow became divine nectar sent to answer their prayers.

At best it was a minor victory. Despite their efforts, it was becoming clear that they hadn't prepared for the harshness of Arizona's extremes. They would make it through the next two years only by grace. They were convinced that their budding powers would be enough to keep the elements at bay.

Christie McNally still seethed at the way Roach had summarily removed her from power. She wanted to reach out to her followers and respond to the allegations that she and Ian were mad or unstable, so she scrawled a note on loose-leaf paper. As her pen worked its way across the pages, the writing grew into a teaching that was five thousand words long and included a spirited reference to Christie's favorite film. It was called "A Shift in the Matrix," and she wrote that it was a teaching meant "to dispel the darkness by shining light." Curiously, throughout the thirty-three-page letter, Christie referred to her husband as Ein—a new name for a new beginning.

She knew that too many people were scared that the couple was in the throes of an abusive relationship. She wanted to reexplain how she came to stab her lover.

My Love was learning how to deal with being in a relationship with someone who had a lot more power than him. At the beginning it was difficult, and he broke down on occasion. It was all divine play to me, really, but these breakdowns were devastating for my poor husband. Because after all, I am also his Lama. So we prayed together to everyone we could think of for help, including Kali.

Kali, she implied, answered their prayers. They weren't engaged in combat; rather, the stabbing was a final act of catharsis that expunged the remnants of Ian's violent nature. The violence was actually a great miracle. His karma ripened as the goddess Kali, in the guise of Christie, stabbed him three times. He emerged a better and more peaceful person.

The sacrifice of his body was an indication of his total surrender to his lama's authority. It was after the event that Christie learned to see Ian as her own divine teacher.

One of the highest Tantric vows there is is the vow of how you should see your Lama, and how to behave towards Them. When you are with a partner, your partner becomes your highest Lama. So I have been Ein's Lama for many years, but he recently became mine as well. Your Lama is unquestionably a divine Being and your job at all times is to fight any desire to see Them in a lesser way. You should trust your Lama with your life, and totally surrender to them.

The politics of mutual surrender are complex, but living as they were in isolation, there was a sort of poetics to it. Entrusted with each other's spiritual progress, they also relied on each other for day-to-day existence with their fates joined in lockstep. Outside this small, rocky safe haven, the rest of the world scorned their choices. It was up to her to set the outside right. Christie claimed that she could access a sort of truth that no one else could. "I have attained certain realizations, and nothing anyone can do or say will change that."

Despite that, she wrote that her expulsion had forced her to attempt to reconcile the earthly realities with the spiritual ones; the politics of Diamond Mountain reeked of a bad divorce settlement. When she and Roach failed at eternal love, the shock wave of their breakup rippled through the community. She blamed Roach's tantric lusts for the discord among the retreatants.

I feel like people have started taking the practice of Tantra too lightly—it is not some recreational activity you do for fun, it is a path to enlightenment, and it is a fast path and very dangerous if misused. People have all sorts of wild ideas that maybe they will start practicing Tantra and have a dozen consorts, or something like that. They enter in for the wrong reasons, and abuse it, and get hurt. Or they try to practice sincerely, but are misinformed, and fail.

The board of Diamond Mountain was reckless, she charged, as she worried that in their haste to remove her from leadership, they set her up to fail at completing her remaining two years of meditation. "You don't just throw someone from deep solitude straight into the crazy world. And we were given no time to prepare a new place to continue," she wrote.

The mistake would have been obvious to anyone who had spent time taking the ACI courses over the last seven years. Delving internally is like diving into the deep sea, where coming up too quickly makes the blood boil in the veins, breaking down the barriers in the body. The mind is little different. Silence allowed the retreatants' minds to expand in new and subtle directions. The strict barriers erected by the board in the valley below were meant to protect them from the outside world. Kicking the couple out so quickly was dangerous. And the board knew it.

Why, she asked, would they threaten to call the sheriff? Did they want her to go mad? Casting her out, she said, was no different from the baseless accusations that ignited the war with the Apache. "They accused the Apaches of stealing [a] child, and this started a 75-year war, a war that, quite honestly, still hasn't healed. The same old battle seems to keep being perpetuated. But perhaps this time we can do it with wisdom and heal this place for good."

The letter seethed with paranoia. At night she heard voices and footsteps outside her tent. She watched searchlights comb the valley floor. They had a good view of the retreat valley from their perch, and she reported that as she and Ian watched from the top of the bluff, people searched their former meditation hut and sealed its doors so they couldn't get back in. Perhaps, she mused, they wanted to find "incriminating photos of a certain ex-friend of mine," possibly referencing illicit photos of Roach dressed in women's clothing, which have never surfaced but have been rumored to exist.

The letter ended on a hopeful note, although, crucially, it also revealed their location. She wrote of her and Ian sitting in their idyllic meditative cave tucked in a sleeping bag and gazing over the retreat valley. It was important for her that the retreatants know she was still sitting above them. All they had to do was look up and they might see her. Then she wondered what would happen to the beautiful and strife-filled land before her.

On the twelfth of April, Christie handed the note to one of her attendants, probably Chandra, who found them during a supply run. Two days later, Akasha posted it online and it was an instant beacon to Lama Christie's followers. The moment of triumph lasted only a few hours before the paradise that McNally and Thorson were both trying to visualize began to crumble down around their ears.

Almost immediately after her attendant left, McNally felt the woozy instability of her guts clenching up. She doubled over in pain and the sickness progressed quickly. She crawled into the cave and within a few short hours was too sick to get up from her place on the futon. Ian worried next to her and did what he could to keep her comfortable.

A light snow fell on their campsite on the night of April 15 and the powder collected in the basin formed by their tarp. McNally's attendant hadn't resupplied them with fresh water when he picked up the note, and the moisture came like a blessing. The next day the temperature coasted above freezing and the tiny melt drained into their eight-gallon jug. Though Akasha had given them a water filter for just this sort of emergency, the couple refused to use it. After all, water was the stuff of life, and purifying the water with their minds—even in the face of McNally's sickness—seemed well within their capabilities.

Whether it was dysentery, an amoeba, or some other bug, the sickness took on a significance beyond the mundane. "The people at the hospital hypothesized that we may have gotten sick from something in the snow, but I don't think so. . . . It was the day after I delivered the letter that I got sick. Now is that a coincidence? Maybe. Maybe not. That is all I can say," she wrote later. Though she didn't expand on the thought, she connected the release of her public statement to her diseased body. The only person she would believe had the power to bring on such an illness was Michael Roach, a man to whom she'd made a lifelong commitment as her lama. Was it possible that Roach planted a karmic seed for retribution? Had Roach and the board set up the couple to fail, not just out of negligence but out of actual malice?

Whatever the cause, Ian was concerned. He trekked down the fifty-foot slope to the cave where they stored their things to retrieve what clean water remained in their stash. There wasn't much—a jug at most—and bringing it back up the hillside, even though it was a short distance, was a treacherous scramble over loose gravel. Unable to fend for herself, Christie trusted Ian with her life, as she'd professed in countless teachings. It was all she could do. They had no antibiotics, antidiarrheals, or other medicines. Ian stayed by his wife's side and lent whatever aid he could with his presence. His mind may have lingered on the cell phone and SPOT locator device that Akasha had given them, but calling for outside help was anathema to their mission. It was her karma to be sick, and his to bring her back.

Ian's energies dwindled from the stress. Over the years, his body had gone through many transformations. He would quit eating and diminish, only to later come back to food with gusto. When they'd lived in the valley below, he'd verged on an ascetic frame almost as a breatharian might. Or perhaps as an anorexic. Now his ribs protruded through his skin like a ladder, and fleeing into the mountains had only worsened the situation. Since they'd come here, neither he nor Christie had eaten fresh food. The tastiest meals in their stores were cans of split pea soup, and the lone bag of basmati rice offered only minimal nourishment.

Later, Christie remembered that "Ian was taking care of me. We had water but not so much, and we were rationing—a couple bowls a day. Ian could have gone and gotten more, but he did not want to leave me. We could have texted someone, but Ian wasn't so keen on people knowing where we were. And, as I discovered, even if you describe the place it was still almost impossible to find."

After nearly eight days of withering away, Christie began to mend. The pall of sickness pulled back and she felt energy slowly creep back enough that she could stumble out of the cave. As she got more mobile, Ian began to feel the same symptoms that she had.

It is easy to underestimate how severe the toll of dehydration can be. In the three years prior to this, thirty-six people died of dehydration in Cochise County. Moisture is at a premium in the desert, and when compounded by something that makes your body lose fluids quickly, like giardia, the situation can become deadly much faster than in civilization. Ian crept into his bed and shivered. He was weak, but not willing to give up.

Christie wasn't made for the outdoors in the same way Ian was. She hadn't hiked and scrapped across mountainsides. Just recovering herself, she was too weak to haul water up from down below to help Ian replenish his lost liquids with anything other than the increasingly brackish water at the bottom of the jug.

A week since the last snowfall, the jug brimmed with twigs and debris. On the twentieth, Ian was pale and worn. His parched lips cracked and dry bits of skin flaked off. It was frustrating and Ian had no one else to blame for his predicament but himself. Sickness was a symbol of his own failure, and he knew that the only way to recover was to overcome whatever karma had caused the illness.

Since he fell back under the sway of Roach in Germany, Ian had taken out his aggression on women in his life. He and Christie had fought in the retreat. But now, on the mountaintop, he turned his aggression inward. They argued over something and then Ian bashed himself on his head with his hands and then with a rod of hardened plastic that they had with them in the cave. There was anguish and failure. And dry tears may have streaked down his cheeks. The bout of rage lasted until Christie begged him to stop.

A bruise swept across Ian's forehead. It wasn't his fault that nothing made sense anymore: The laws of karma are never straightforward. Christie knew that the cause of illness isn't ever linear. Bacteria might deliver a fever, but the set of conditions that allowed the bugs to colonize his body descended from his earlier deeds. Karmic sickness was as dangerous to their mission as bodily disease. In their cosmology, sickness is not always a bad thing. Karmic seeds can ripen only once, so every pain that Ian suffered helped purify negative things in the past.

Christie knew that when Ian looked out of the cave at her with the fading light of his eyes, all he wanted to see was her as an angel made of pure white light. Christie McNally was his lover and his lama, the enlightened being who had seen the nature of emptiness directly. Whatever happened next, he had surrendered his fate to her. He had absolute faith that she would do the right thing.

When he fell unconscious, the responsibility to bring her husband back to health rested solely on Christie's shoulders.

Her choice was to use the SPOT beacon and accept that fate was out of their control or help purify her husband's karma and pull the

sickness out by its root. She didn't require much deliberation. Mc-
Nally could see her husband's rage and frustration and asked Kali for
help to bring him back from the brink as she had before. A book she
kept in the back of the cave had a cover illustration of the emaciated
goddess holding a severed head. It rested next to a sacred drum that
they used for their rituals.

Dysentery was an unforgiving mistress; over the course of two
long and brutal days, the bacteria ripped its own path through Thorson's digestive system. The stench of filth must have filled up the
dank cave. His physical resources depleted, he hovered on the verge
of life and death.

Would he recover as she had? Or would this journey kill him?
McNally prayed and fell asleep while Thorson shivered beneath layers of blankets, his ribs and hip bones protruding up through his skin,
his lips chapped red with dried blood.

On the morning of April 22, 2012, Thorson did not wake up.
McNally's prayers hadn't worked, and consequences pierced her reality. She could still make out the slow rattle of his breathing and
worried that perhaps now he was beyond her powers. At six a.m.
she activated the SPOT locator beacon and sent out a prerecorded
message that indicated her GPS coordinates to her friends and family. The signal pinged a satellite in geosynchronous orbit above the
earth and ricocheted it down to an emergency service center in
Houston. McNally also fired up the cell phone and texted Chandra
down below. She told her attendant that Ian was breathing only
shallowly and that she wanted help. What's more, she needed deliv-
erance from her own decisions.

Back at Diamond Mountain the developing emergency brought
the community together with a flash of responsibility. Her attendant
told Scott Vacek that McNally and Thorson were nearby and that
they needed help. Diamond Mountain threw together a search party
to locate the former retreat leaders and headed up the mountainside.
Renee Miranda, the nurse who had originally stitched Ian's wounds,
came out of retreat to assist. Vacek called 9-1-1, and search and rescue
scrambled a helicopter from the nearby air force base.

The terrain that protected Thorson and McNally from discovery also hindered their rescue. The search party toiled up the mountainside for six hours before they reached them. Miranda was the first to see Christie's terror-stricken face. By now, Ian was no longer breathing. His face had an unnatural deep purple sheen. Miranda felt for a pulse and told her former lama that Thorson was gone.

"That single moment will forever be the worst moment of my life," McNally wrote later.

An hour later a helicopter rigged for mountain rescue sliced across the open range and over the spot where Thorson lay. There had been mechanical difficulties on the way, which explained why they arrived after the crew that hiked up the mountain on foot. Miranda and Vacek used a red sleeping bag to signal the chopper to their exact location.

Rescuers rappelled down from the side of the aircraft wearing a special harness called a screamer suit and hauled McNally to safety. The officer took several photos of Thorson's corpse and began recording the details for a police report. In the photos, Ian holds his hands over his sternum in graceful repose. Sand silted over his eyes and a dark bruise arched across his nose. The diamond earring that he wore to symbolize his link to the goddess Vajrayogini reflected brightly in his right ear, and his gold wedding ring balanced loosely on his finger as if ready to fall off. His mouth hung agape, leaving an open space where his last breath had slipped away.

McNally screamed at the rescuers to save him, even though his corpse was all that was left. In the sheriff's report a ranger recorded her saying, "I thought they could bring him back." McNally did not want to be separated from his body and fought the police and mortician with fists and tears when they tried to take it into custody.

An autopsy eventually attributed Thorson's death to dehydration. His corpse weighed only one hundred pounds. McNally recuperated in a hospital in Willcox and was treated for dehydration. As soon as she was able, she went to the mortuary to sit next to Thorson's body and hold his hand into the afterlife.

Two days later, Kay Thorson received a knock on her door. She

looked through the peephole and saw the security officer for her
building shifting on one foot to the other with an anxious look.
When she opened the door, the officer handed her a phone number
for the sheriff's station in Willcox, Arizona. The feeling of dread
seemed to creep up from the floor itself and she knew that Ian was in
trouble. Probably hurt.

When she rang the sheriff, Larry Noland, his words seemed to
pass over her as if they came from a distant reality. She hadn't heard
any news of her son since he walked off into the desert, and now information seemed to rush in without a break. There had been a stabbing. A cave. In the next few days, there would be a funeral.

Akasha arranged the memorial service at Christie's behest. When
Kay called, he promised to manage all the details necessary to bring
her out to Arizona. She left on a Friday and flew into Tucson and
drove across the valley between the Dragoon and Chiricahua mountains, where Akasha had booked her a room at a characterless hotel
by the highway.

Ian's casket lay in a low prefabricated funeral home called West-
lawn Chapel. Kay wore a black dress. Only one other person from
Ian's family attended: His ten-year-old daughter, Thea, flew in from
Germany without her mother.

The coffin gaped open during the ceremony, which the funeral director said was a remarkable feat since McNally had refused to let him em-
balm the corpse. Her memory hazily settles on McNally reading Buddhist
scriptures and offering the corpse white silk scarves as a blessing.

McNally read a short Buddhist scripture on the perfection of wisdom that Roach had translated for her years before. The scripture
dwelt on the emptiness of death.

*There is no misunderstanding your world. There is no stopping this mis-
understanding, and the same is true all the way up to your old age and
your death, and to stopping your old age and your death. There is no
suffering. There is no source of this suffering. There is no stopping this
suffering. There is no path to stopping this suffering.*

The passage was almost nihilistic, grim and meaningless. Like Ian's life, it passed too quickly. For Kay, it was a small tribute for her son and she wished there had been more about the man she remembered rather than the one that he had become.

When it was over, Kay had only one request. She wanted to understand why her son chose to come here. What was it about Diamond Mountain that was so special? She wanted to see the mountain with her own eyes.

Kay asked Akasha, who then asked McNally for permission to visit the Buddhist campus. Diamond Mountain was only twenty miles away, but McNally told him to keep her away. So Akasha told Kay that it would be impossible and that she wouldn't be welcome there. Kay asked again, but the answer was the same. They wouldn't take her, not even to an overlook from Fort Bowie.

"I knew they were lying, but I didn't think I should just show up there alone," she said.

So instead, Kay struck out on her own. She zeroed in on a small mountain just outside of Willcox that looked out across the desert town. The only landmark on the side of the mountain was a giant white W meant to identify the name of the town to any traveler who came through the desert. It wasn't the place she wanted to go, but she hoped it would be enough to get a sense of the land that inspired Ian.

The hike was deceptively brutal. What looked like an easy climb from the base of the valley grew steep when she got near. She leaned heavily against the incline of the ascent and had to stop to catch her breath every few feet. It took all morning, but when she finally stood at the top, she could see that the land extended endlessly in all directions. To the west, the formidable Chiricahua Mountains guarded the entrance into Apache Spring. It was barren, and in places the range seemed to be little more than piles of boulders stacked on top of one another. It was desolate and unforgiving country. As the wind wicked the moisture from her lips, she knew she could never forgive the people who took her son from her.

Epilogue

White Umbrella Protection

You can ask [a member of the Zande tribe about the cause of a man's suicide] "How did he kill himself?" and he will tell you that he committed suicide by hanging himself from the branch of a tree. You can also ask "Why did he kill himself?" and he will tell you that it was because he was angry with his brothers. The cause of his death was hanging from a tree, and the cause of his hanging from a tree was his anger with his brothers. If you then ask a Zande why he should say that the man was bewitched if he committed suicide on account of his anger with his brothers, he will tell you that only crazy people commit suicide, and that if everyone who was angry with his brothers committed suicide there would soon be no people left in the world, and that if this man had not been bewitched he would not have done what he did do. If you persevere and ask why witchcraft caused the man to kill himself the Zande will reply that he supposes someone hated him, and if you ask why someone hated him your informant will tell you that such is the nature of men.

—E. E. Evans-Pritchard,
Witchcraft, Oracles, and
Magic Among the Azande

THERE IS NO TRAIL to the cave where Ian Thorson died. It sits on a loose gravel slope somewhere above the valley. When I first reported this story, it took me three hours scrambling upward over a steep slope and loose rubble, and past mean-looking cacti and poison-tipped yucca to reach it. The journey almost killed me. When I ran out of water, something just shy of heatstroke made my movements sluggish. I spent the bulk of the day recovering from the climb and talking to a few of the personalities who hung around the valley. That night I crawled into the tent that I'd pitched in one of the washes around Diamond Mountain. It was a hot and windless night, so I removed the fly so I could see the sky through the mesh roof.

A million twinkling points of light pierced through the dark blue ether above me. Perhaps I was simply exhausted by the long day, but as I sat there looking at the sky, it seemed to me that the colors began to shift. The sky turned from a deep darkness into a deep pink and finally a red hue as if it were an organic thing with its own will. I wondered if my eyes were playing tricks on me, if the rods and cones were realigning themselves with heightened aware-ness. But, I have to admit, part of me wondered if there was more to Roach than showmanship. The people at Diamond Mountain spent their lives trying to bend the material world to their own will. De-scriptions of *siddhis* have filled sacred texts for more than two thou-sand years. Several of my sources claimed that Roach could work miracles, and now I was on Roach's turf, writing a story that might not be very flattering. I wondered what it would mean if Ian had died not because of ignorance and dysentery, but because Roach had planted a bad seed into his karmic stream? The thought was crazy, so I let it go.

It took nine months from when I first reported it for the story to appear in *Playboy*. In that time, Diamond Mountain's relationship to journalists changed drastically. Articles that were critical of the group ran in *Psychology Today* and on a raft of websites and in tabloids. Mc-Nally came into the public eye only once, when she sent a writer at *Rolling Stone* an almost sixty-page screed about her relationship with Roach. Members of the group who once enthusiastically embraced a chance to set the record straight began to shy away from the lime-light as headlines focused on tantric sex, alcohol-infused orgies, and dark rituals. Almost everyone who had intimate knowledge of Thorson or McNally went quiet, perhaps at the behest of Roach. The inner circle was essentially closed for business.*

As Diana Alstad and Joel Kramer predicted in their book *The Guru Papers*, Diamond Mountain had entered that stage of fringe religious movements when they turn inward and feel persecuted by the society at large. According to their scheme, when this happens, finances begin to dry up and it becomes increasingly difficult to attract new members. Roach wrote Fernanda Santos at *The New York Times* asking her to publish a clarification that downplayed Thorson's death, saying that "since the article came out, our charity—which is one of the main sources of income for Tibetan refugees—has lost a number of donors." The next stage, according to Alstad and Kramer, predicted that the group would begin stockpiling weapons and see outside criticism as a serious threat. This worried me.

There was still more to the story, and I knew I would have to go back to Bowie in 2013, when the remaining retreatants planned to come out of the valley for the first silent retreat teachings since Ian's death. (Quiet teachings were scheduled every six months or so for a total of six over the course of three years.) At the same time that Diamond Mountain seemed to close off, estranged members were con-

---

*Over the course of researching this book, I made several attempts to ask the leadership at Diamond Mountain to respond directly to various contentious statements and documents that I uncovered. Michael Roach refused to speak with me in private or respond to my e-mails on three different occasions. When I completed the manuscript for this book, I sent a list of fifty questions to Roach that I thought might be particularly controversial. His personal attendant, Elly van der Pas, a nun whom he ordained with the name Jigme Palmo, and the longest-serving member of the Diamond Mountain Board, responded to me as follows:

When the press first started to show interest in what happened in the federal land next to DM, friends who were familiar with the press advised GMR not to say anything. But he felt he had nothing to hide and gave a number of interviews, mostly through e-mail. Of course he was taken aback when what he said was taken out of context, or ignored, or otherwise twisted to make him out to be some kind of villain, and the opinions of a few ex-students who had no first-hand knowledge were given equal or more weight.

Most of the questions you are asking have no bearing on Ian's story. Most of them are attempts to confirm what seems to be speculative hearsay, or assumptions based on hearsay, or just irrelevant. There is no answer—the premise is wrong. Try to put yourself in his place. You might try to set the record straight for a while, but if that does no good, why continue to waste your energy?

People will assume what they assume. There is nothing GM can do to change that, apart from trying to continue to act positively to make good things happen in the world and understand that ultimately nothing bad can come out of that attempt.

—Elly van der Pas (Jigme), June 7, 2014

tacting me in droves. Many people were angry at Roach for his idiosyncratic Buddhism. Monks at the FPMT, one of the largest organizations of Tibetan Buddhists in the West, wrote that they were glad the truth was coming out. Several ex-members were convinced that the cause of Ian's death wasn't only his encounter with the elements, but that he was a victim of black magic. Among my correspondents were monastics at Roach's former home base in New Jersey, people living on the land near Diamond Mountain, and a former attendant to Lama Zopa of the FPMT, named Karen Visser, who claimed that I, and other journalists, were targets of spiritual warfare.*

Visser was a tenacious correspondent with journalists, sending me more than two hundred messages, and countless more to the other reporters as they observed the decline of Diamond Mountain. Shortly after I first started reporting on Roach in 2012, she called me to say that the highest lamas at Sera Mey had offered to cast a protection spell that would protect journalists and their friends from Roach's karmic meddling. I declined the offer for two reasons. First, I worried that it might unduly bias my reporting. And, second, I wasn't inclined to think that anyone, let alone Roach, had special powers. Visser was surprised I said no; other journalists accepted.

Half a year later I began work on this book. I accepted a spot at a writer's retreat in upstate New York called Ledig House and planned to outline the project. I would have a year or so to complete the manuscript, and my first action when I arrived in New York was to send an e-mail directly to Michael Roach, asking him to reconsider his policy of not talking to me. I told him that my drive to understand Ian

---

*In my days as a graduate student in anthropology in Madison, Wisconsin, I had a chance to study under the late professor Neil Whitehead, who wrote the classic book *Dark Shamans Kanaimà and the Poetics of Violent Death*. That work explored the terrifying world of *Kanaimà* shamans who ritualistically stalked and murdered their victims over the course of several years. Kanaimàs believe that increasing the terror their victims feel will give the shamans the sacred powers of the jaguar. Whitehead wrote, and frequently talked about, how he suspected he had been cursed by a shaman during his fieldwork in the Guyanese jungle. A sickness came over him that no Western doctor could treat. He was at death's door and had to be carried out of the wilderness by porters. It was only after he met another shaman in the city of Georgetown who made him drink a bitter potion that the illness retreated. Whitehead was continually fascinated by that event and, sometimes, seemed a little terrified. He died unexpectedly young while I was working on the manuscript for this book.

Thorson's life was also a way of making sense of my former student who took her life at the Boot Institute in Bodh Gaya: the same place where Roach lectured at the turn of the millennium and began his affair with Christie. I wrote, "I have often puzzled over the meaning of [Emily's death], wondering if I should take the last words she wrote in her journal—I am a Bodhisattva—as a serious spiritual revelation, or whether they were a sign of madness. Perhaps it could have been a little of both." The e-mail went unanswered, and I could only wonder what Roach might have thought of it.

After I reached out to Roach, everything in my world began to come unglued with a suddenness that would have been familiar to Christie McNally after she handed off her letter "A Shift in the Matrix" to her attendant. The picturesque grounds of the retreat—the place where I finished my first book three years earlier—took on an ominous air. My small room painted gray with a double bed was a simple writer's space with a desk and a place to stash my clothes. There were two windows: one above the bed and another that looked out over the driveway. Within a day or two of sending the e-mail to Roach, I noticed that a single wasp had taken a habit of hovering over my pillow. Since I don't much like killing insects, I would get up from my chair and shoo it out the window. But whenever I closed the window, another wasp would show up within ten or twenty minutes. An insect was always over my pillow. Never anywhere else in the room. Their persistence was commendable. There must have been thirty or forty of the bugs over the course of the two-week retreat (or perhaps it was just one very indefatigable wasp, circulating from outside to in). I got into a routine where I would begin working and look up to see a recently expelled wasp watching me.

In Tibetan Buddhism, different deities are often associated with the presence of animal or insect life. For instance, the deity Dorje Shugden, who the Dalai Lama calls an "evil spirit," is said to send spiders out to people he is interested in. I wasn't sure if wasps represent any specific deity, but once they started showing up regularly, I felt what I can only describe as a presence. I began to also see things out of the corners of my eyes. There was a human-size black oblong object that resembled a large hairy amoeba that always seemed to be just outside my field of vision. If I got up from my desk to walk outside, the shadow would hang there at the limit of my field of view. I'd turn to look at it, but it would disappear. Its presence didn't frighten me, exactly, but it always seemed to be around.

For me, writing is an immersive experience and I knew that I had to get deep and inhabit, as much as possible, the mental space of my characters. To do that, I transcribed my former student Emily's journal, transmuting her bubbly script into the digital files native to my computer. As I typed, I played various talks that Michael Roach had posted freely online. The process connected me to the material in a way that was probably not healthy. I was getting paranoid. The constant presence of wasps rankled my nerves.

And it got worse with time.

There was a strange tingling at the base of my skull, and a sort of heaviness not unlike a clogged sinus, only it was in the wrong area of my head. Writing was difficult. A slew of grants that I applied for months earlier to help me finish the book came back with rejection letters. I checked the balance of my bank account only to discover that cyber thieves based in Nigeria had gotten hold of my debit card and bought more than a thousand dollars' worth of schwag in foreign countries. When I called my wife in California, things were not going well. My marriage was deteriorating. None of this was, of course, something I could blame on Michael Roach in any sort of rational way. But I was becoming a student of the irrational. I sent Visser an e-mail saying that I had reconsidered her offer for protection. It was probably all just bad luck and paranoia, but I was seeing a pattern in the coincidences and a little extra mojo couldn't hurt.

The most worrisome aspect for me was that I planned to visit the upcoming quiet retreat teaching in Bowie roughly a year after Thorson had died. The event was coming up in a few weeks. While I didn't think Diamond Mountain was going to turn into Jonestown or Waco, it was impossible to predict how some members might react to a threat to their community. One of the most important vows in the pink books that people at Diamond Mountain carried around was to prevent threats to the *sangha*, which is the Sanskrit word for religious community. According to several accounts, there were automatic weapons at Christie McNally's Kali initiation.

Certainly they would be praying that whatever bad press I might cause would go away. I knew that if I were ever going to be in spiritual trouble, it would be then. So I agreed to buy tsampa—a sort of barley flour—for the monks at Sera Mey as an offering. In return they would conduct a powerful ceremony known as the white umbrella protection puja. Visser told me that the spell would permanently forge a connection between me and their highest lama, a very old and spooky gentleman named Khensur Rinpoche Rabga. She wrote that "this is shamanistic protection, old stuff, some of it predating Buddhism. Tantra itself goes back to the Paleolithic." It seemed good enough for me to justify the $210 it would cost for eighty monks to chant a protection spell in my name for a few hours.

Diana Alstad once explained to me that the nature of a guru's power works like hypnosis: You can be affected by it only if you have already invited the guru into your mental space. It's a notion akin to the old myth of vampires being able to enter someone's house only if they've received an invitation. Although they don't tend to comment on what might happen in the divine world, anthropologists have long known that magic has real-world effects even if the underlying causes could be purely psychological. Fetishistic magic and shamanism alter people's behavior and can serve to explain complex cultural structures. A person who thinks he is cursed might indeed experience a bout of negative events. Whatever was causing my symptoms—paranoia or the hidden weave of karma—I knew I had to kick Roach out of my head. So I made up my own meditation. There was no real method except focusing my mind with the intention of booting out bad juju.

A wasp buzzed over my head as I faced the window. I took long deep breaths, imagining that every inhale was positive light filling my body, and I exhaled the black mist of Roach's influence. I began to rock back and forth in my chair for no discernible reason. Almost immediately, I felt a rush of energy coming up from my stomach to my head. It was like a heaviness being lifted. I breathed in positive energy and expelled the muck that had been collecting at the bottom of my skull. The relief was remarkable. As the meditation came to a close, my computer pinged an announcement of a fresh e-mail. I looked up and glanced at it; it was from another journalist who had been working on a story about Roach. She said that she had given up on her project and wanted to send me all the notes she had in case I wanted to make sense of it all. It seemed that obstacles were clearing up.

There were still two days before I planned to head out to Diamond Mountain, first on a flight to my home in Long Beach, California, and then the eight-hour drive across the Sonoran Desert to the mostly abandoned town of Bowie. My spirits were up and I went to meet some of the other writers in the kitchen. Among them was Robert Karjel, a Swedish military officer and author who was working on a thriller about his service flying helicopters around the world. I told him that I planned to spend my time on Diamond Mountain land and he wrinkled his chin and warned me to take precautions. He told me to be aware of where the exit was, no matter where I was sitting. I should identify people in the room and make an escape plan if necessary. It was military mumbo jumbo, but I appreciated his concern. And then he said something that really worried me. He recommended that I carry a knife. It wouldn't be for self-defense, but because if I was sleeping in my tent and someone had an intention to harm me, I would be vulnerable. A knife would let me slash the nylon and get to my feet.

The advice echoed of the Bascom Affair, or "cut-the-tent" as the Apache remember it, when Cochise escaped certain death at the hands of a foul-intentioned Union army lieutenant. Cochise slashed through the wall of the tent and escaped into the same mountains where McNally and Thorson would spend their last days together a century later. I wondered if I might need to do the same as Cochise had. I told Karjel I would keep a knife with me at least when I slept.

The wasp was gone when I went back to my room. Soon I was on my way to Cochise County. After I landed in Long Beach, I jumped into my car and flew past endless miles of stately saguaro cacti and empty desert valleys. When I was on the road, Karen Visser sent me another e-mail, which pinged on my iPhone. The monks had completed the puja, and she sent me a long protection mantra. I scrolled through the ancient syllables.

hrih benza krodha hayagriva hulu hulu hum phat

I parsed the words slowly over my lips and worked them around my mouth. They were foreign, and strange, but saying them helped calm my nerves as I bolted down the highway. I committed them to memory and repeated them a half day later when I rolled down the long dirt road from Bowie to the Chiricahua Mountains for the second time.

I parked in the lot amidst a couple dozen other cars. Standing off to the side was a security man with a buzz cut and a poorly fitted suit. He stayed by his car with a wire arched up, over, and around his ear. The first person I saw whom I recognized was Scott Vacek, the man who had become the public face of Diamond Mountain and was responsible for day-to-day public relations. He said I was welcome to attend the event and offered me a smile that seemed genuine. But the era of open access was clearly over. The members of the so-called inner circle who had known Thorson avoided me and frowned when I got near. Attendees wore T-shirts that read SPIRITUAL GANGSTER and shuffled uneasily when I scribbled notes in my pad.

It was uncomfortable to be there, but I didn't feel I was in danger. If anything, they were scared of me and what I might write. In the evening, Roach arrived in a white minivan. Mercedes Bahleda, dressed in a flowing black dress, marched in front of her teacher with a dour expression. Her eyes opened wide like saucers when she saw me. As Roach passed he looked into my eyes and smiled hello and said, no, he still wasn't going to talk to me.

So we shuffled into the temple and sat down for the normal ceremonial rounds of meditations and floral dedications that were part of the routine at Diamond Mountain. The talk seemed to go on endlessly. One speaker after another ranged over mundane administrative topics. The board of directors fund-raised for a new expansion for a kitchen and student center to a room divided by a high curtain.

Sometime earlier in the evening the retreatants filed in unseen and entered the room through a separate entrance. They sat in the silence to which they were accustomed and listened to the dharma lecture. Roach took the stage exactly one year and one week after Thorson died. He didn't acknowledge the anniversary. Instead, his talk seemed to verge on the apocalyptic. Diamond Mountain wasn't the only place under stress, he said; the world itself was in trouble.

> There will be major social problems. There will be violence, there will be wars, there will be starvation, no roads, no packaging, no asphalt, no fuel for ships. Everyone else is crazy. You are the only sane ones. When I see this university I see something totally different than what the rest see. You are a shining light in the world. . . . There are no physical limitations or political limitations if you have that worldview because it comes from seeds in your mind.

He seemed to swell on the stage. A hint of anger crossed his face as he examined the way Diamond Mountain was getting a reputation as a dangerous fringe group. At one point he turned back to the importance of maintaining an altar every day in order to keep a focused mind.

> Putting out an altar isn't a hippie thing to do, it is an advanced thing to do; you are extremely intelligent. I don't care what anyone else says. They are crazy. They will live and die without any meaning to their life.

Roach's was the last lecture of the evening and it was pitch-black outside when his talk was over. He asked people who were involved in his tantra class to meet him at the Lama House, but everyone else could have the night off. Some people piled into cars headed for hotel rooms in Willcox. Most everyone else had tents. I brushed my teeth in the communal bathroom and walked slowly to my tent. I'd set it up in the wash as far as possible from the temple and anyone else's campsite.

It was a small tent from REI that was really only big enough for one person but could technically hold two. I lay on my back, going over the events of the evening and worrying about what might happen if I heard footsteps crunching up the gravel path. It wasn't a quiet night like the one a year ago. Wind funneled through the narrow walls of the valley and shook the thin fabric of my tent, which in turn swayed and bobbed in the currents. Sudden gusts kicked the stakes out of the sandy ground and the rain fly flapped madly in the air like a flag on a battlefield. As the nylon sheets rubbed against each other, sparks from the static electricity danced across the ceiling. My knife was within reach, and I kept my sleeping bag open enough so I could get up in a hurry if I had to. It took a long time, but I eventually fell asleep. I dreamed of Michael Roach.

In my vision I was somehow standing above Roach on a ridge or staircase, looking downward at him. He glided forward as if his feet were not touching the ground. There was a sort of sinister intent in his face and as he drew closer he attempted to make eye contact. About three feet away, just before our eyes met, I felt something pulling me toward him. It was as if a hand had grabbed my shirt and yanked. It was hard to breathe. I was suffocating. Before we touched, I managed to wrench myself awake. There was a storm outside and the walls of the tent billowed concave from the force of the wind. It pressed against my face like a sail. My heart raced in my chest with steady thumps.

Several sleepless hours later the sky outside was a deep blue. The dawn couldn't be too far off. I said the mantra and waited for the sky to slowly brighten. The dream shook me.

I spent much of the next morning hiking in the foothills around the valley. I climbed up one round top where I'd been told the Apache had burned a $15,000 offering to clear off the bad spirits from the land. I found the remains of a campfire at the summit, but not much else. The hill offered a good view of the surrounding mountains and valleys. I sat down and waited, figuring I could get a view of the retreatants as they made their way down from the closed valley above.

After about a half hour, two people in all-white outfits walked down from the valley along a dirt path that runs parallel to the main

road. They entered the back door of the temple for a morning meditation. I couldn't make out any details except to see that they kept a
slow and steady pace. After I'd scanned the hillside, my eye fell onto
a small green cylinder lodged between a slab of granite and the
ground in front of me. I reached down and pulled up a brass shell
from a military carbine. The casing bore the date 1878, which meant
it would have been fired toward the tail end of the war that cleared
the Apache from the valley. I was getting used to seeing patterns in
the events around me, and I wondered whether the shell sat here for
a hundred and thirty years unnoticed specifically so I would pick it
up. Or perhaps it was only litter from a forgotten time, and chance
explained how it ended up in my pocket just as well as anything else.

I descended from the hillock in silence and waited in the room for
the retreatants to come from behind the curtain. It was the first time
any of them would have used their voice in more than a year. There
were several speakers—the retreat leader who had taken over for Mc-
Nally as well as people who had once sat on the board of directors.
Most were circumspect. None offered thoughts on what happened to
Thorson.

Then Lobsang Gyeltse—a fifty-ish woman in maroon nun's robes—
climbed onto the stage from across the thick curtained divide. She
wore a pink blindfold to shield her eyes. She took a seat on the same
throne that Christie McNally had occupied when she disclosed the way
she had stabbed her husband. The nun's voice was careful and contemplative, if also a little sad. Sometimes she peeked beneath her blindfold
to glance at index cards she had prepared for her speech.

She said that in the retreat, meditation had slowed down her perception of the world. As McNally had said a year before, Gyeltse likened her own realizations to the film industry. She had begun to see
her mind as a sort of movie camera that conjured up images of the
world that were both essential and meaningless. What the mind did
best was to organize those images and create a narrative. "The story
we are most fascinated with is our own story. But what is this story?
Am I my story?" she asked. "These projections are responsible for my
physical world, but also my mental world. I see pictures of myself in-

teracting with the world. Our goal is to find the cause of suffering and pain. In retreat I'm trying to change the pictures." She then quoted the poet Muriel Rukeyser: "The universe is made of stories, not of atoms."

Gyeltse's face shone with lucidity. Part of me scoffed at the disassociation with material reality. At the same time, I knew she was also partially right. I had come here to tell a story of Ian Thorson and, to some degree, Emily O'Conner. Telling their stories had changed me. I took on their traits. Their lives instructed the way I saw the world. Did it matter whether it was paranoia or karma that made me so nervous? Did it matter that I felt better after I'd prayed in a language that I did not understand? Roach sat on a cushion in the front of the speaker, and I thought about how most of the people here saw him as a man on the cusp of enlightenment. Around the country many people saw him as a charlatan bent on manipulating his followers for his own gain. Could he be both at the same time?

I thought back to the only time that Roach had ever truly addressed me. It was a year earlier as I made my way back to Los Angeles from Diamond Mountain with a day stopover in Phoenix. Thorson had been dead for only a month and the community was still grappling with the loss. I'd come off the mountain wondering how it was possible that Christie McNally hadn't simply pressed the button on the beacon a day earlier and saved Ian's life. I wanted to ask him what he thought. Roach was teaching *lamrim* that evening. It was the same series of texts I had listened to in Bodh Gaya before Emily took her own life. That evening's talk was on the importance of mindfulness. It lasted three hours, and when he was done, I got in line behind a fifty-ish Indian woman who was carrying a Louis Vuitton handbag. She chatted with other people in the line, examining a necklace of beads that she hoped her guru would bless. "I can't believe I'm going to meet the Enlightened One," she said excitedly.

When it was my turn I stood in front of his throne in the New Age church and introduced myself. I tried to phrase a question about how he was dealing with Thorson's death. He began to talk. "It was a very sad event, but why are people not interested in my teaching? One person dies in the desert and suddenly everyone pays attention. People should be talking about all the good works that I've done instead." He then waved me away and promised to respond to me in writing, though I knew he never would.

It wasn't a satisfying answer. It was as if Roach couldn't take a minute to reflect on the profundity of what had happened. To him it may just have been karma ripening, and perhaps the story didn't end when someone died in the desert. It might have just begun.

In March 2014, the thirty-four remaining retreatants walked down a dirt road after a thousand days in the desert. They approached a gate with two boots nailed to its posts, which demarcated the farthest-most limit of the *tsam*. Before they crossed the threshold, the group set up a small folding table and placed sweet cakes and cookies on it as an offering to the spirits of the valley. As they lowered their heads in prayer, a heavy gust of wind shot down the ravine and coated them in dust. When they were done, Michael Roach emerged from the crowd of well-wishers and greeted them with a bouquet of roses.

In the three years that the retreatants meditated on visions of a perfect world, the planet did not seem more peaceful than it did before. That morning, I read news that reporters had been gunned down in Afghanistan as they covered a new round of elections. In another story, search crews were giving up hope of ever locating an airliner that went missing somewhere between Malaysia and Beijing. I wondered how Roach's acolytes would take the news.

It was the third time I came to visit the valley and my second retreat teaching. My real reason for coming, though, was not to see the retreatants but to understand the place where Christie and Ian stayed for more than a year, now that the grounds were open to the public. It was a long walk up past the dried-up creek and parched riverbed, but when I made it to the Lama Dome, where Ian and Christie had spent their year in retreat, the sandstone tiles on the porch were loose and shifted below my feet. After they left, someone had installed an iron security door to protect the entrance of the house from intruders. After Ian died, the board elected to leave the spiritual center of the retreat abandoned, its secrets locked behind foreboding doors.

Termites burrowed holes into the beams that held up the roof and front porch. Paint peeled off the balcony where the couple once assumed yoga postures together. At one time, any retreatant could look up from their cabin and see Ian's and Christie's arms and legs entwined in a dance of love and enlightenment. If the retreatants' gaze continued in a straight line to the mountain behind the valley, they might have been able to make out the ridge where the two of them spent their last days together.

I sat on their porch swing for a while and wondered what the future might hold. Christie McNally had disappeared and mostly been silent since Ian's death, surfacing for only a single media interview. Still, rumors skittered through the community that she was in either Bermuda or New York planning her comeback. Some people still saw her as their lama. One day, perhaps she'll have more to say. Perhaps there are still spiritual lessons to learn.

Farther down the valley, in the temple, Michael Roach was entertaining a Chinese investor named Ming Feng Wu who had flown in from Beijing. They'd hit it off on one of Roach's world tours and Wu promised to deliver the next round of funding for Diamond Mountain. He'd pledged $1 million to construct a new student center, and Roach was prodding him for more cash to construct a second ACI dharma center in Sedona, where he could continue to teach tantra courses.

Later that evening, Wu would give a lecture on mind-only Buddhism and how someone could cultivate wealth with the power of karmic seeds. The scandals that rocked the Diamond Mountain community in the United States had less impact on its global reputation. Crowds still flocked to Roach's lectures in Asia, Europe, and South America.

I peeked in the windows of the Lama Dome and tried to see the place where Christie and Ian worked out their karma at the point of a knife. It was surprisingly clean for an abandoned building. Diamond Mountain announced plans to rent out the space in the coming years

to other religious groups who want to run their own meditation retreats. Roach envisions that perhaps he'll be able to attract business
leaders to study in Arizona and teach them ways to guarantee their
future wealth. They will come here for weeks or months at a time to
delve into the emptiness of their minds. Only the curious will learn
what happened here.

Notes on Sources

THIS IS A work of nonfiction. As with any endeavor that attempts to reduce the infinite complexity of the world into the written word, it is also the work of an author with his own biases and limitations. Though I have used people's real names, there are a few sources whose identities I felt it was important to protect and have thus changed their names and relevant details. There are a few places in the text where I attempt to understand the perspective of a particular character during their private prayers and meditations in a way that would be clearly impossible without the ability to commune with the dead. In these moments, I have reconstructed what the routines would have looked like through the commentaries of experts, students, course materials from Diamond Mountain, and advice from longtime meditators. When quoting sources directly, either from letters or from taped recordings, I have often opted to fix grammatical errors and confusing diction for the sake of clarity. In all cases, I have aimed to preserve the intentions and meaning behind the words. These are stylistic decisions for which I hope my readers may forgive me. The following notes are an attempt to allow my readers to re-trace the steps I took to bring the story into book form.

Author's Note

Emily O'Conner's journal as it appears on pages xv and 235 is perhaps the most haunting document I have in my possession. Just thirty-three pages long, it documents her first moments in India to what may well have been her very last thoughts and sentiments. It came into my hands during the police investigation into her death. It has never been published in its entirety, and I suspect that it never will be.

Prologue: The Cave

I culled together the time line for McNally's and Thorson's last days in the cave from primary and secondary sources. Several police reports filed in Cochise County and Ian's postmortem examination mention several wounds on Thorson's body, his meals, and the approximate time of death as well as snippets of conversations between law enforcement and the people on the mountain that day. When search and rescue arrived on the scene, the officers took dozens of digital photographs of the cave and of Thorson's body with his arms crossed over his chest. McNally's own note, "A Shift in the Matrix," which was published online at scribd.com, gives a peek into her mind the moment before she fell ill, and the eerie sense of paranoia that pervaded the retreat valley at the time. Chandra, who asked to be identified only by his Tibetan name, helped fill in the remaining details based on his memory of McNally at that moment.

PART ONE: ENLIGHTENED MINDS

The First Bodhisattva: A Buddhist Parable

This story has been recounted dozens, if not hundreds, of times in the Buddhist canon and in lectures in monasteries around the world. As with the other parables in this book, this is my own re-creation of those events.

Chapter One: Enlightening America

The opening epigraph to this chapter is generally attributed to the revered Tibetan sage Padmasambhava. However, as Paul Hackett notes in his 2008 PhD dissertation at Columbia University titled "Barbarian Lands: Theos Bernard, Tibet, and the American Religious Life," it is at best a paraphrase of what Padmasambhava said. I have used it to open this chapter to draw a distinction between what we hope is ancient Buddhist wisdom and what we can actually verify. Which is to say: not very much. Perhaps the most accessible and best-written account of how selective our understanding of Tibetan lore actually is, is Donald Lopez's *Prisoners of Shangri-La*, to which I am forever indebted since I first encountered the book as a college student. Also informing this discussion is Catherine Albanese's *A Republic of Mind and Spirit*, which catalogues America's curious fascination with mystical thinking, as well as *American Veda* by Philip Goldberg. Less critical of the movement of Tibetan ideas to the West is Sogyal Rinpoche's 1992 *The Tibetan Book of Living and Dying*, which is probably the preeminent contemporary example of magical teachings of Tibetan Buddhism. Excellent accounts of the Dalai Lama's escape from Tibet can be found in his autobiography, *Freedom in Exile*, or in Heinrich Harrer's 1952 classic, *Seven Years in Tibet*.

Chapter Two: The Box

As the title of this chapter indicates, almost all references about Ian's early life derive from the box of materials that he gave to his mother before he set out for Diamond Mountain. In addition to those several thousand journal entries, receipts, ACI course materials, letters, and hand-drawn maps, I had the great fortune to interview several of Ian's family members and childhood friends, who, in some cases, furnished me with correspondence and memories of Ian as a young man. I spent several days interviewing his mother, Kay Thorson; his grandmother, known as Gagi; and his sister, Alexandra Thorson, in New York. Among the people he knew in high school and college, I spoke with his girlfriends Fernanda Hannah and Ceren Osmanas well as Mike Oristian and Saul Kato. The esoteric works mentioned in this chapter include José Silva's New Age classic *The Silva Mind Control Method* (New York: Simon & Schuster, 1977), and a book by Alexandra David-Néel that Ian read on the road but never mentioned by title. However, people interested in David-Néel's biography might enjoy reading *The Secret Lives of Alexandra David-Néel* by Barbara and Michael Foster (Woodstock, NY: Overlook Press, 1997).

Chapter Three: The Curious Prehistory of Michael Roach

Michael Roach is fond of recounting his life story, and various versions of it can be found on his website, in his book *The Diamond Cutter*, which he coauthored with Christie McNally, and in numerous open letters he has published on open forums. Furthermore, videos and transcripts of lectures he has posted on YouTube.com provide the bulk of my understanding of Roach's formative years as well as his own accounts of his high realizations. Numerous Internet forums by ex–Boy Scouts detail the secret ceremonies of the "Order of the Arrow." His first employer, Ofer Azrielant, confirmed the details of Roach's employment, while multiple sources spoke of internal controversy about the cover of the book *Preparing for Tantra*. (Interestingly, however, others denied it ever happened.) Roach's book *The Garden: A Parable* offers another account of Roach's first encounters with a young lover of his who, he realizes, is also the goddess Vajrayogini. Amnesty International published a report on conflict diamonds, while an excellent exposé about the trade's connection to Surat ran in Jason Miklian's article "Rough Cut" in *Foreign Policy*. C. J. Chivers provides a vivid account of the movement of arms from former Soviet stockpiles into the hands of the world's most notorious militant groups in his riveting chronicle of the history of the AK-47, *The Gun* (New York: Simon & Schuster, 2010).

Chapter Four: The Acolyte

Palden Gyatso's stories are a matter of public record and his full testimony is available from the Office of Tibet (tibetoffice.org). Accounts of the Tibetan Freedom Concert come from media reports from the time and my memory of watching it on MTV as a teenager. Other accounts of the concert's popularity are in Donald Lopez's book *Prisoners of Shangri-La*. Descriptions of the early days of the Three Jewels come from current and former ACI students as well as online transcripts, some of which can still be found on the website michaelroachfiles.wordpress.com. Information from Christie McNally's early life comes from her book *The Tibetan Book of Meditation* and from interviews with several of her college friends, most notably Ara Babajian. The murder of Mercedes Bahleda's mother, Renee Bahleda, comes from contemporary newspaper accounts in *The Daily Gazette* and *The Sun and Erie County Independent*. When asked directly whether her parents were murdered, Bahleda claimed that my account was "not true." When confronted with the press clippings she responded "no comment." The quote from Christie McNally describing what it meant to take a root lama came from T. Monkyi's interview titled "Interview with Geshe Michael Roach and Christie McNally" from Easter 2003. Michael Roach delivers his lecture on the emptiness of a pen at just about every open forum he attends. While I do not have a transcript of the actual inaugural lecture, the quotes in this section derive from his 2013 book *The Karma of Love* and a lecture titled "Using a Flamethrower to Cut Your Nails," which Roach delivered on

October 31, 1997. Very similar quotations can be found in any number of transcripts published on the ACI website theknowledgebase
.com. Accounts of his lectures were also found in Ian's notes along
with several letters to and from LaShaun Williams.

Chapter Five: Programming

The description of Kay Thorson's preparation of Ian's breakfast is
something of a composite of the meals I had with Kay and her personal descriptions of how Ian changed after he began attending lectures at the Three Jewels. The description of Ian's personal meditative
experiences derives from conversations with several current and former Diamond Mountain students, Ian's letters, Remski's descriptions,
and tantric teachers outside of Roach's lineage, including Sati Ah, a
tantrika and yogini in Long Beach, California. Yet it should be noted
that due to the personal nature of meditation, it is only my best attempt to understand the imponderabilia of his mind. To some extent,
writing this raises the crucial question of what constitutes nonfiction.
Or, for that matter, what is truth? It is my belief that this section is a
true account, even though I am treading into a world that I could
never absolutely know. Copies of Roach's "The Book: Make Your
Dreams Come True" are available at most of his public lectures and
for free online. Anthony A. Simmons, then director of the Root Institute, did not respond to my inquiries directly; however, his reactions
to Roach were recorded on the anti-Roach blog michaelroachfiles.
wordpress.com. The transcript of Ian's Bodhisattva vow ceremony
was generously provided by Kay Thorson.

Chapter Six: Deprogramming

The opening quote for this chapter comes from Matthew Remski's
post on *Elephant Journal*, titled "Psychosis, Stabbing, Secrecy & Death
at a Neo-Buddhist University in Arizona." This blog post initiated
most of the media attention in Ian Thorson's death and expertly

delved into the unusual tantric practices that Michael Roach taught to his followers. The books *Snapping: America's Epidemic of Sudden Personality Change* by Flo Conway and Jim Siegelman and *The Guru Papers: Masks of Authoritarian Power* by Joel Kramer and Diana Alstad have emerged as the most influential works in anticult literature. I've had a chance to interview the authors and was repeatedly referred to these books by Kay Thorson and the exit counselors she worked with while arranging Ian's intervention. Other than these references, most of the descriptions from this chapter emerge from primary sources left by Ian in the box and from interviews with direct witnesses. There was some disagreement about whether or not Ian jumped out of the window of the Roosevelt Island home—at different times Kay Thorson remembered that he simply used a back door, and Joe Kelly clearly remembered a window exit. All sources agreed that the intervention put Ian in an erratic state of mind.

Chapter Seven: Diamond Theosophy

Stephen Batchelor's *Confession of a Buddhist Atheist* recounts his own years as a Buddhist monk in different traditions. I spent an afternoon skyping with Batchelor about his memories of Michael Roach when they both studied in Dharamsala. His book deftly explores how little we know about the Buddha's life after enlightenment. This chapter relies mostly on secondary historical sources, including works that I've already mentioned, by Donald Lopez and Catherine Albanese. Of course, any student of anthropology will notice the influence of Edward Said's classic *Orientalism* in the discussion of the transmutation of ideas between East and West, as well as Nicholas Dirks's classic *Castes of Mind* for his analysis of the spread of Indic languages. Interestingly enough, Michael Roach has dramatized the way Tibetan texts were translated, in his novelization of a translator's journey titled *How Yoga Works*. More scholarly approaches can be found in Ronald Davidson's *Tibetan Renaissance* (as quoted in this chapter) and Douglas Duckworth's article "De/limiting Emptiness and the Boundaries of the Ineffable." In *Tibetan Renaissance,* Ronald Davidson offers a more complete description of the philosophical differences between Dolpopa and Tsongkhapa:

> [In Dolpopa's] tradition, ultimate reality is pure and unchanging. It is the noumenal world of a metaphysical reality, an absolute reality that is "empty" in the sense that it lacks all that is other—all the unreal, impermanent phenomena that comprise the deluded world—but this ultimate reality is not empty of itself; it is the ineffable ground of reality. . . .
>
> The Geluk tradition consistently argues that the ultimate truth is necessarily a mere absence and nothing more; it should not be treated as another substance. According to their tradition, emptiness itself is empty; thus, it has no real referent and is certainly not a metaphysical presence that is above and beyond phenomenal reality. Rather emptiness simply means the absence of inherent existence in any particular phenomenon.

There are hundreds of excellent works on early Buddhist saints and the theoretical arguments that shaped the course of the religion. The most colorful character in the book is probably the phallophilic Tibetan saint Drukpa Kunley, whom I learned about in Georg Feuerstein's *Holy Madness* and Keith Dowman's *The Divine Madman,* from which the excerpt on page 105 was taken. Given the ribald nature of Kunley's poetry, it is likely that the translator of this particular poem substituted the words *thunderbolt* and *lotus* for *cock* and *pussy* to tone it down for readers in English.

Readers interested in learning more about the roots of Madame Blavatsky's theosophy might check out the aforementioned works by Lopez and Albanese, or Gary Lachman's *Madame Blavatsky.* The Theosophical Society's mission statement is drawn from page 50 of Philip Goldberg's *American Veda: How Indian Spirituality Changed the West,* as well as additional reference to page 336 of Albanese's *A Republic of Mind and Spirit: A Cultural History of American Metaphysical Religion.*

Theos Bernard is the subject of two recent biographies by Paul Hackett and Douglas Veenhof. The two accounts use the same basic information to tell two radically different stories. Hackett's book, based on more than a decade of research during his PhD coursework at Columbia, is a scholarly dissection of Bernard's lifework—at times showing how important he was to the development of Tibetan studies, but also highlighting the underlying charlatanism. Veenhof's begins with a tribute to Geshe Michael Roach and extols Bernard's mystical abilities and tantric teachings. Veenhof refused to comment when I contacted him. Multiple sources have suggested to me that Michael Roach may consider himself a reincarnation of Theos Bernard.

The battles of the Himalayan Plateau are detailed in Peter Hopkirk's *Trespassers on the Roof of the World: The Secret Exploration of Tibet* (London: John Murray, 1982).

Chapter Eight: Skillful Means

The opening poem in this chapter, Michael Roach's "Letter to My Lamas," was originally posted on the Diamond Mountain website but was hastily taken down once it became controversial. However, very little ever truly disappears online, and there are several blogs dedicated to preserving the wrong turns that Roach and other prominent Buddhists have made. I have spent many hours reading through the collected archives at buddhism-controversy-blog.com and michaelroachfiles.wordpress.com. Amber Moore, Allison Dey, and Sid Johnson all gave me accounts of their time on the first retreat, as did many other people I engaged on my travels back and forth from Arizona. Susan Howler, who was one of the original retreatants with Roach and McNally, spoke to me initially, and retracted various parts of her account once I mentioned the allegations posted on the blog geshe watch.blogspot.com about possible sexual liaisons. The letters between Roach and the Dalai Lama are still part of public record and published on the official website of His Holiness, though I had to rescue Lama Zopa's response from a very deep part of the Internet. I was also able to similarly retrieve official transcripts of the first Great Retreat teachings in 2003 from the Diamond Mountain website before they were taken down. And although to this day I have been unable to discover any information about the mysterious journalist T. Monkyi, who interviewed Roach and McNally about their spiritual experiences after they left the first Great Retreat, I am forever indebted to whoever preserved the full transcripts of his interview and archived them publicly.

PART TWO: SACRED SPACES

The Buddha and the Ferryboat

This parable was first told to me by the Dutch guru and extremophile Wim Hof. At the time, I was working on a different story for *Playboy* and he used the parable to explain the difference between miracles and his spirituality. I've found further references to the tale in Somerset Maugham's novel *The Razor's Edge* and in Edward Conze's *Buddhism: Its Essence and Development*.

Chapter Nine: Sacred Spaces

The opening quote for this chapter comes from page 70 of Keith Basso's "Wisdom Sits in Places," which I first came across in a graduate student seminar. Basso's essay was in an anthropology volume called *Senses of Place,* which showed me many of the ways that different cultures conceive of the land around them. As I researched this chapter, I read deeply, perhaps *too* deeply, into Apache religion and history and cut much of what I discovered out of the final manuscript. The second quote that opens this chapter comes from the best book, by far, about the history of the U.S. conflict with the Chiricahua: David Roberts's *Once They Moved Like the Wind*. Roberts chronicles the lives of both Geronimo and Cochise in elegant detail, and the book is well worth exploring on a lazy Sunday afternoon. Most of the quotes about the history of Apache Pass come from this book. I am also indebted to anthropologist M. E. Opler's 1930s accounts of the Apache belief system, the best known of which is *An Apache Life-Way*. I discovered geological information about the Chiricahua Mountains in literature published by the National Parks Service. I first learned about the shoot-out at Miracle Valley from the Cochise County sheriff, Larry Noland, who brought it up in relation to Ian's death. The only book I could find on the subject was the rather disappointing *Shootout at Miracle Valley* by William Daniel. Daniel's book tends to skew toward the perspective of the police officers involved in the shoot-out and lacks voices from the church itself. I learned about the sacrifice to the Apache god Ussen from Ekan Thomason as well as from postings about it in the Diamond Mountain archives.

Chapter Ten: Twelve Years, Fifteen Feet

Christie McNally's opening quote in this chapter comes from Nina Burleigh's article in *Rolling Stone*, "Sex and Death on the Road to Nirvana"; she has been the only reporter to date to interview McNally after Ian Thorson's death. Their correspondence included an almost sixty-page manifesto from McNally, and Burleigh generously shared excerpts from that document with me. I have used several quotes from it throughout this chapter and in later chapters. I had the great privilege to speak with the Tibetan scholar and geshe degree holder Robert Thurman over the phone while first reporting this story. His meeting with Roach at his office in New York in 2003 has become something of a legend among Diamond Mountain aficionados—a confirmation that Roach's teachings made a serious break with Tibetan orthodoxy. At the time of this writing, the legal case against Michael Gordon, the founder of Bumble and Bumble, has still not settled, though Gordon remains free and, presumably, in New York. The indictment by the IRS was made available to me through their public relations department, and when news of the arrest was made public, almost all reference to Gordon on Roach's various websites disappeared. The book they wrote together, *Karmic Management: What Goes Around Comes Around in Your Business and Your Life*, is still available on Amazon. Chronicling the years that Ian Thorson spent in Germany proved to be a reporting challenge. In those years Ian mostly stopped communicating with his family in New York, leaving only a few records behind to explain the sudden violent shift in his personality. His girlfriend, Beatrice Steimer, refused to extensively comment for this book, forcing me to rely on a few work connections, Fernanda Hannah's memories, and a lengthy police report filed in Berlin. Details about the construction of Diamond Mountain were much easier to come by: For one, I interviewed the board of directors at Diamond Mountain, most notably Jigme Palmo, Rob Ruisinger, Nicole Davis, and Scott Vacek. Other people who witnessed the construction of Diamond Mountain were Michael Brannan, Ekan Thomason, Sid Johnson, Allison Dey, and one source who wishes to remain anonymous. I have heard descriptions of Michael Roach's high school girlfriend from three sources at Diamond Mountain but decided to redact her name. I decided to leave out several other allegations of Roach's love interests—including a twenty-ish model from New York and a nun—from the final text since I was not able to independently confirm them, and, frankly, I thought it would divert the narrative. Mercedes Bahleda and Eric Brinkman (Nyingpo) gave me a lengthy interview together while we were in Phoenix but neglected to mention that they were married. I learned of the story of their arranged marriage from several people who attended the ceremony.

Chapter Eleven: Ian and Christie

Kay Thorson recounted to me the story of Ian and Christie's trip to the Sivananda Retreat Center in the Bahamas based on her son's telling of it to her around the time of their wedding. Ian's previous relationships were often talked about among people at Diamond Mountain, but it was difficult to find any single individual who would give a sustained narrative of his time in Arizona. Since Ian either stopped recording his thoughts, or his writings mostly disappeared, this chapter includes my best understanding of his time there. My specific sources are mentioned in the body of the chapter and have been cited in other sections of these notes. Anna Wheeler, the mother of Ian's second child, refused to comment; however, many of the people close to Ian have left digital trails online. I obtained divorce records of Roach and McNally through the Yapavai County Courts, and their marriage records from Fernanda Santos of *The New York Times*. Photos of Thorson and McNally's marriage are available on the website Flickr.

Chapter Twelve: Exodus

To solicit donations for the second Great Retreat, the board of Diamond Mountain launched the website retreat4peace.org, which included links to various blog posts by prospective retreatants and to videos of retreat leaders. One fund-raising video shows Thorson and McNally walking away into the night as they begin their vow of silence. Another video, posted on YouTube, recorded McNally's farewell speech with the title "Lama Christie's Talk to Retreatants' Families." I was able to retrieve many similar documents before they were taken offline. Understanding the context of how McNally came to stab Thorson was very important to the goal of this book, and the entirety of her speech was almost immediately taken down and exists in the hands of only a few people high up in the Diamond Mountain hierarchy. However, after the event, the board asked Renee Miranda to file a statement with the Cochise County sheriff about what she witnessed, and in that report was an excerpt from McNally's public talk. Whoever transcribed it did so word for word and included McNally's peculiar Southern California syntax. I removed at least thirty *likes* and *ums* from the excerpt to preserve clarity. While I don't have a hard record of the rest of the speech, I spoke to several witnesses who could recollect the context. Since Thorson's death, Diamond Mountain has released numerous statements online, including an official open letter penned by Michael Roach on their website diamondmountain.org as well as several rebuttals to Matthew Remski's account on elephantjournal.com. There are a further two or three thousand comments on the threads, which can suck any persistent researcher down a never-ending rabbit hole of Buddhist in-fighting. I had a lengthy conversation with Akasha, one of McNally's attendants who arranged her flight into the mountains and helped establish a time line for events. Michael Brannan was one of the last people to see McNally before she left (albeit almost a month before Ian's death) and he provided me with a handwritten transcript of their conversation, which was preserved because of McNally's vow of silence.

PART THREE: THE DARK NIGHT OF THE SOUL

The Suicide Sutra: A Buddhist Parable

I first learned about the existence of what I have termed the Suicide Sutra in the wake of my student Emily's death in Bodh Gaya. A Buddhist scholar with whom I had studied as a graduate student told me that during the Buddha's time many students committed suicide. The parable originates in the Pali Vinaya in the story of Migaland-ika. The best account I have found of this parable outside of the original is in Liz Wilson's scholarly work *Charming Cadavers*. Other versions of the story have appeared in sources as diverse as the *American Law Review* and various dissertations on Buddhist ethics. While most ac-counts focus on how the Buddha declared Migalandika a "sham re-cluse" after the spate of murders, it seems apparent that at least some of the responsibility for the mass deaths lies with the Buddha's rather extreme teaching. It should be noted that Tibetan Buddhists still teach a practice called chöd, which centers around meditating on de-caying corpses. A similar practice is common among Hindu ascetics and is known as the Aghori. Technically this story is not a "sutra," which is a word that denotes that it came directly from the mouth of the Buddha; rather, since it is from the Vinaya, it is considered a later commentary. I hope that readers will indulge my preference for allit-eration in this instance.

Chapter Thirteen: Spiritual Sickness

The challenge for this chapter was to try to connect the tradition of diagnosing spiritual sickness in meditative traditions with credible scientific research. Amy Cayton's book *Balanced Mind, Balanced Body: Anecdotes and Advice from Tibetan Buddhist Practitioners on Wind Disease* was an entry point because it attempted to translate the idea of *lung* for a Western audience. Of course, the tradition of esoteric literature identifying meditators who fell off the spiritual path goes at least back to the time of the Buddha. In the West, cautionary tales began to arrive only after the hippie revolution of the 1960s. Gopi Krishna's *Awakening of Kundalini* is a modern classic for both identifying and warning about the possible dangers of kundalini experiences. As more Westerners became disillusioned with Eastern techniques, legal cases like *Kropinski v. M. M. Yogi* became increasingly common. While reviewing those proceedings, I was initially surprised to see my uncle Keith Wallace's name mentioned, which in turn opened a little-talked-about chapter in my family history. Wallace's original research is easily located in the journal *Science*, as are the thousands of other meditation-related studies that followed his pioneering work. I am very encouraged by the ongoing research by the neuroscientist Willoughby Britton, whose work on problematic experiences during meditation can be found on her website brittonlab.com. Other excellent talks by her have been posted on the website buddhistgeeks.com. In the winter of 2012, I spent several days in her lab at Brown University listening to her own profound and occasionally disturbing meditative experiences. The second half of this chapter mostly derives from an article I published in *Details*, titled "Death on the Path to Enlightenment," where I trace cases of several spiritual seekers who went missing in India. The *Journal of the American Medical Association* study referred to is by Madhav Goyal et al: "Meditation Programs for Psychological Stress and Well-being: A Systematic Review and Meta-analysis." The Australian Qigong-induced psychosis study is detailed in Beng-Yeong Ng's "Qigong-Induced Mental Disorders: A Review." Finally, the psychiatrist Meredith Sagan introduced me to the concept of "spiritual bypassing."

Chapter Fourteen: Death on a Mountainside

Almost two years after Ian Thorson's death I am still astonished by the existence of the gray seed pot that he and McNally found in the cave. I spent an inordinate amount of time trying to identify its uses and origins. Mike Jacobs, archaeological collections curator at the Arizona State Museum, ultimately identified it as either Hohokam or Mogollon extraction. Daniel McGrew, who works for the Bureau of Land Management, is currently the pot's custodian at Safford, Arizona. Establishing the time line of events that led to Thorson's death required cross-referencing McNally's own published statement, "A Shift in the Matrix," with weather reports kept at Fort Bowie, the coroner's report, and numerous police filings, as well as interviews with Diamond Mountain board members, Sheriff Larry Noland, and McNally's attendant Akasha. Emergency personnel photographed the interior of the cave and Thorson's body before they removed it. I was also able to track down the funeral director who oversaw Ian's final ceremony and see a record of the event that he kept.

Epilogue: White Umbrella Protection

I chose to begin this chapter with a selection from E. E. Evans-Pritchard's classic work *Witchcraft, Oracles, and Magic Among the Azande* because it underscored how supernatural explanations of causation have existed in one form or another since the beginning of recorded history. Since Evans-Pritchard's time, we know that magical explanations occasionally work—oracles sometimes herald future events, and people who believe they've been cursed sometimes experience bad luck—but we can never truly know whether the cause is external and mysterious, random chance, or a reflection of human psychology. To some degree it may not matter. This chapter derives entirely from my own experiences steeped in stories and documents from around Diamond Mountain. I will leave it to the reader to decide what it means.

Acknowledgments

No book is ever truly the work of just one person. The months of sweat, dedication, and imponderable details would simply have been for naught without the generous support of a community of editors, agents, sources, and experts. Most important, I am indebted to the family of Ian Thorson, who generously supplied decades of his handwritten notes. Kay Thorson met with me in her family dining room over the course of several sweltering summer days on Roosevelt Island and allowed me a peek into her family's life. It seemed fitting that a portion of the royalties for this book would be contributed to a fund to support the continuing education of Ian's two children.

Charlie Conrad at Gotham Books has seen the project through from its infancy, and I have benefited greatly from his calm editorial hand. My literary agent, Laura Nolan, helped me revise a sprawling draft of the original story into a potent proposal. Also at Paradigm, Katelyn Dougherty and Jason Yarn oversaw endless legal details. My film agent, Judi Farkas, helped me think of my characters in new ways.

I would never have gone to Arizona were it not for an afternoon phone call from my editor at *Playboy*, Stephen Randall. Every publication in New York and San Francisco rejected the piece when I brought it to their door, but Stephen told me to start driving east and send him something brilliant. Shane Singh, the fact-checker, made sure that I got all the details correct. Great thanks are owed to Jesse Ashlock, formerly of *Details*, who oversaw my article on spiritual sickness. And Colette Davidson, who interviewed a source in France for me.

Over the years, I have enjoyed support from the Schuster Institute for Investigative Journalism at Brandeis University, where I am a senior fellow. There, Florence Graves, Melissa Ludtke, Claire Pavlik Purgus, Elizabeth Macedo, and Neena Pathak all weighed in on different parts of the project. Students at the institute, including Michael Haskell and Zachary Reid, helped sort through the box of materials left to me by the Thorson family and double-check the time line of events. In addition, Baptiste Jacquemet designed my website and Karrah Beck revamped my graphics.

While reporting is often a competitive venture, with journalists fiercely patrolling their leads for exclusive information, my experience on this story has been entirely different. Fernanda Santos of *The New York Times* generously shared volumes of material that I would otherwise have never found on my own. Nina Burleigh, who wrote a piece for *Rolling Stone,* was the only reporter to actually speak with Christie McNally after Ian's death. She shared parts of the transcripts with me. Both Jennifer Beyer and Jesse Hyde wrote their own stories, which I was able to reference in the course of my reporting. Anna Schecter of ABC and I shared notes about our time on Diamond Mountain.

As with my first book, I wrote a portion of the manuscript in the idyllic New York countryside at a writer's residency called Ledig House. There I shared wine and literary conversations with DW Gibson, Anna Moschovakis, Rama Sangye, and Mathilde Walker Clark, and they witnessed me worry about my upcoming return trip to Diamond Mountain.

I have been fortunate to have long conversations on Buddhism and modern India with a wide variety of generous and patient souls. Among these is my friend Jason Miklian, who read an early draft of the manuscript and convinced me to cut the parts that were dragging it down. A yogini, real estate investor, and tantric teacher, Sati Ah, whom I lived with in Long Beach, California, helped flesh out my understanding of deep meditative experiences and fill in some of the blanks of what Ian Thorson may have been experiencing. Padma Govindan helped me think through the story for several years and gave deft editorial guidance about what I needed to cut from the original article. My debt is deep to her. Also weighing in were Daniel McNamara, Christine Karwoski, and scholars Tenzin Bob Thurman, Paul Hackett, Matthew Pistono, Willoughby Britton, John Dunn, Meredith Sagan, Rachel McDermott, Amy Cayton, Diana Alstad, Joel Kramer, and Stephen Batchelor.

I also benefited from the wise counsel and perception of numerous people who intimately understood the inner workings of Diamond Mountain and spiritual sicknesses. In no particular order these people included Ekan Thomason, Michael Roach, Matthew Remski, Kay Thorson, Alexandra Thorson, Gagi, Fernanda Hannah, Saul Kato, Mike Oristian, Karen Visser, Susan Howler, Michael Brannan, Sierra Schafer, Tenzin Peljor, Nicole Vigna, Scott Vacek, Jigme Palmo, Sera Mey Monastery, Gregory Tranchina (of the IRS), Claudia Engel, Collette Davidson, Jyotsna Singh, Amber Moore, LaShaun Williams, Gaya Police Thana, Joe Elder, Rick Ross, Patrick Ryan, Joe Kelly, Bill Zavatsky, and Joel Guyton Lee.

I've also enjoyed the counsel and support of other writers and journalists who have weighed in on different parts of this process. My thanks go out to Yudhijit Bhattacharjee, Brendan Koerner, Ransom Riggs, Graeme Wood, Jonathan Green, Sarah Spivack LaRosa, Brooke Hauser, Sarah Topol, Benjamin Skinner, Akash Kapur, Randy Dotinga, Erin Siegal McIntyre, and E. J. Graff.

In June, I walked into the offices of my agency in New York with an urgent request to scan several thousand documents in just a few short hours. Sara Schlievert, Dan Stebbins, Marissa Loil, and Rebecca

Henning jumped into the task and should be recognized with more than the cupcakes I repaid them with. At Gotham Books I was also fortunate to have levelheaded advice and reviews by Matthew Martin, as well as copy editing by Joy Simpkins, and assistance shuttling the manuscript through production by Leslie Hansen.

Of course, my family has also stood by me through the entire insane process of writing a book. My mother, Linda Carney; Wilfred Carney; Joan Carney; Laura Carney; Allison Carney; Rosie Ettenheim; and Sage Hopkins: I love you all. And thank-you to Dan and Mara Carney for putting me up in Phoenix every time I stopped through on my way to another trip into Cochise County.

Finally, special thanks to Laura Krantz, who read and reread my problematic chapters until I got them right. We spent a long Fourth of July weekend in Idaho with her family poring over manuscript corrections together, missing out on the wilderness adventures we'd planned. She brightens my life every day that she is in it.

Glossary

Andin International—a successful jewelry company where Michael Roach worked for more than a decade. It is now owned by Warren Buffett.

Asana—a yoga posture, often done in sequence

Asian Classics Input Project (ACIP)—an effort to digitize and preserve Tibetan texts, a project founded by Michael Roach with a grant from Hewlett-Packard

Asian Classics Institute (ACI)—an institute founded by Michael Roach to teach his own brand of Tibetan Buddhism

Atman—a Hindu word for an essential self, or soul

Avalokiteshvara—the Tibetan god of compassion. The Dalai Lama is said to be the earthly incarnation of this deity.

Ayurveda—an ancient Hindu medicine system

Bardo—the intermediate state between death and rebirth

Bhagavad Gita—a Hindu epic in which the Lord Krishna discusses the nature of karma and dharma with the warrior Arjuna

Bodh Gaya—the village where the Buddha attained enlightenment

Bodhichitta—the mind of a Bodhisattva, which Buddhists attempt to emulate

Bodhisattva—a divine being on the verge of enlightenment who chooses to stay in the world and help all sentient beings also become Bodhisattvas

bodhisattva—a compassionate person who helps others

Buddha Nature—latent potential that resides in all sentient beings, which, if developed, will lead them out of suffering

Chakra—a spinning wheel of energy inside the subtle body

Chöd—meditation on decaying corpses

Consort—a deity's partner during tantric practice

Dakini—a carnivorous feminine spirit

Dalai Lama—the temporal and spiritual leader of the Gelukpas, and, more broadly, Tibetan Buddhists. The current Dalai Lama, Tenzin Gyatso, is the fourteenth in the succession.

Dharma—religious duty

Diamond Cutter Institute—an organization founded by Michael Roach that uses Buddhist teachings for success in business

Diamond Mountain—a growing complex of classrooms and retreat yurts in the Arizona desert that comprise the center for Michael Roach's organization

Dorje Shugden—a banned Tibetan deity that grants wishes in return for a high price

Dorje Shugden controversy—After the Dalai Lama banned Shugden worship in 1996, Shugden followers murdered the Dalai Lama's teacher in Dharamsala, and since then relations between the two groups have been strained

Drukpa Kunley—a controversial Tibetan saint whose claims of enlightenment let him break many societal norms. An excellent example of the concept of upaya.

Foundation for the Preservation of the Mahayana Tradition (FPMT)—the largest mainstream Tibetan Buddhist organization in the West

Gelukpa—the most powerful and well-known sect of Tibetan Buddhism. They place an emphasis on scholastic learning and knowledge over religious experience.

Geshe—the highest academic qualification for a Tibetan Buddhist; the equivalent of a PhD

Guru—a spiritual teacher. The title is often associated with Hinduism.

Hinayana—literally "lesser vehicle," a now extinct form of Buddhism that included the "mind-only" school

Kagyu—an esoteric lineage of Tibetan Buddhism that stresses retreats and meditative experiences

Kali—the Hindu goddess of death. The name translates literally to "the black one."

Karma—the law of cause and effect in Hinduism and Buddhism where actions from the past determine results in the future after a gap of time—usually over the course of many lifetimes

Karmic seed—a latent karmic action that has not yet ripened into a result

Krishna—a Hindu god with blue skin who lectured Arjuna on the nature of karma and duty in the *Bhagavad Gita*

Kundalini—a feminine spiritual energy that lies at the base of the spine and can be awoken by meditation

Lama—an honorific title for a spiritual teacher in Tibetan Buddhism

Lamrim—a textual introduction to the path to Buddhist enlightenment

Lung (*loong*)—the Tibetan word for wind; also, a disease meditators get that can cause anxiety and, in some cases, psychosis

Mahayana—literally "great vehicle," a later version of Buddhism practiced by Tibetans. Mahayan Buddhists aim to become Bodhisattvas instead of attaining Nirvana.

Mani stone—a stone carved with Buddhist prayers, images, and mantras, often found near monasteries and near the top of mountain passes

Mantra—a word, sound, or sentence repeated during meditation to focus the mind

Mind—the ephemeral thoughts, emotions, and experiences that constitute the self; not to be confused with the bundle of neurons and gray matter of the brain

Mind-only school—a (now uncommon) Buddhist belief that there is no material reality but, rather, that the world is simply a projection of the mind

Momo—a Tibetan dumpling

Mudra—a symbolic hand gesture to symbolize an offering or to evoke a particular visualization

Nadi—a river of energy in the subtle body

Nirvana—the state of enlightenment

Noumenal realm—the world of ideas and spiritual action that are not material reality

Nyingma—the oldest lineage of Tibetan Buddhism

Om—the sound used in meditation or prayer that symbolizes the birth of the universe

Padmasambhava—also known as Guru Rinpoche, an eighth-century Tibetan saint and incarnation of the Buddha

Pali—a dead language in South Asia in which many early Buddhist scriptures were recorded

Prana—energy that connects the subtle body to the universe

Prayer flags—colored flags inscribed with Tibetan prayers, usually hung near monasteries or on mountain passes

Puja—a ceremonial prayer

Rig Veda—the earliest written Hindu text, written sometime between 1700 and 1100 BC

Rinpoche—an honorific title given to the highest Tibetan lamas

Root Institute—the main FPMT center in Bodh Gaya

Sakya—"Gray Earth" Buddhists; the main lineage of Tibetan Buddhism before Gelukpa

Samadhi—the highest level of meditative concentration

Samaya—vows taken by Buddhist initiates

Samsara—the endless cycle of birth and rebirth, which is broken only through enlightenment

Sanskrit—the ancient language in which sacred Hindu texts are usually written. It occupies a position similar to that of Latin for Catholics.

Sera Mey—A Gelukpa monastery whose clergy fled from Tibet and rebuilt the institution in South India. It is part of the great Sera Monastery.

Siddhis—supernatural powers acquired though meditation or yoga and referenced in the *Yoga Sutras of Patanjali*

Star in the East—a teaching institute, founded by Michael Roach, that combines Christian and Buddhist teachings to say that Jesus was a Bodhisattva

Subtle body—the spiritual body of every person, consisting of spinning wheels of energy called chakras, and arterial flows called *prana*, and existing in parallel to the physical body

Sutra—system of ethical laws and teachings that governs Buddhist behavior and is open for anyone to learn

Tangka—a Tibetan ritual painting of a deity that has many secret levels of meaning

Tantra—secret spiritual teachings in Buddhism and Hinduism that require special initiations to study

Tara—a female Bodhisattva of Tibetan Buddhism

Theosophical Society—Founded by Madame Blavatsky, this society was one of the most prolific translators of Asian spiritual texts to the Western world.

Theosophy—an esoteric belief system, which originated in the late 1800s, that combines philosophy with theology. Theosophists aim to discover a universal divine nature by looking for common beliefs across different religions.

Theravada—Sometimes called Hinayana, or "lesser vehicle," Buddhism, it emphasizes perfecting one's own inner Buddha Nature to achieve enlightenment. Theravada Buddhists do not aim to become Bodhisattvas; instead, they aim to achieve Nirvana.

Tsongkhapa (1357–1419)—the founder of the Geluk lineage

Upaya—clever or efficient actions meant to guide students along a spiritual path by someone who has attained high meditative realizations. Also called skillful means, the practice allows the teacher to lie to students if he or she believes that the untruth will lead to greater happiness in the end.

Vajra (also dorje)—a ritual object that symbolizes both a thunderbolt and the male sex organ. It is usually accompanied by a bell, which symbolizes feminine essence.

Vajrayogini—a diamond-like goddess

Vinaya—Buddhist teachings written in Pali that dictate proper conduct for monastics

Yabyum—a position of sexual or cosmic union in tantric practice

Yamantaka—a bull-headed Tibetan god who is called the Destroyer of Death

Yoga—ancient Hindu teachings that join the mind, body, and breath to create a spiritual experience

Yogi/Yogini—male/female yoga practitioners

Bibliography

Scholarly Sources

Albanese, Catherine L. *A Republic of Mind and Spirit: A Cultural History of American Metaphysical Religion*. New Haven: Yale University Press, 2007.

Basso, Keith H. "Wisdom Sits in Places." In *Senses of Place*, edited by Steven Feld and Keith H. Basso. Santa Fe: School of American Research Press, 1996.

Batchelor, Stephen. *Confession of a Buddhist Atheist*. New York: Spiegel & Grau, 2010.

Broad, William. *The Science of Yoga: The Risks and the Rewards*. New York: Simon & Schuster, 2012.

Burleigh, Nina. "Sex and Death on the Road to Nirvana." *Rolling Stone*, June 6, 2013.

Carney, Scott. "Death and Madness at Diamond Mountain." *Playboy*, March 2013.

———. "Death on the Path to Enlightenment: Inside the Rise of India Syndrome." *Details*, October 2012.

———. *The Red Market: On the Trail of the World's Organ Brokers, Bone Thieves, Blood Farmers, and Child Traffickers*. New York: William Morrow, 2011.

Cayton, Amy, ed. *Balanced Mind, Balanced Body: Anecdotes and Advice from Tibetan*

Buddhist Practitioners on Wind Disease. Portland, OR: FPMT Education Department, 2007.

Conway, Flo, and Jim Siegelman. *Snapping: America's Epidemic of Sudden Personality Change*, 2nd ed. New York: Stillpoint Press, 1995.

Conze, Edward. *Buddhism: Its Essence and Development*. Mineola, NY: Dover Publications, Inc., 2003.

Dalai Lama. *Freedom in Exile: The Autobiography of the Dalai Lama*, revised edition. New York: HarperPerennial, 2008.

Daniel, William R. *Shootout at Miracle Valley*. Tucson: Wheatmark, 2009.

Davidson, Ronald M. *Tibetan Renaissance: Tantric Buddhism in the Rebirth of Tibetan Culture*. New York: Columbia University Press, 2005.

Desikachar, T.K.V. *The Heart of Yoga: Developing a Personal Practice*. Rochester, VT: Inner Traditions International, 1995.

Dirks, Nicholas B. *Castes of Mind: Colonialism and the Making of Modern India*. Princeton: Princeton University Press, 2001.

Dowman, Keith, and Sonam Paljor, trans. *The Divine Madman: The Sublime Life and Songs of Drukpa Kunley*. Varanasi, Uttar Pradesh: Pilgrims Book House, 2000.

Duckworth, Douglas S. "De/limiting Emptiness and the Boundaries of the Ineffable." *Journal of Indian Philosophy* 38 (2010): 97–105.

Evans-Pritchard, E. E. *Witchcraft, Oracles, and Magic Among the Azande*. Oxford: Clarendon Press, 1937.

Feuerstein, Georg. *Holy Madness: Spirituality, Crazy-Wise Teachers, and Enlightenment*. Chino Valley, AZ: Hohm Press, 2006.

Goldberg, Philip. *American Veda: How Indian Spirituality Changed the West*. New York: Three Rivers Press, 2010.

Goyal, Madhav, et al. "Meditation Programs for Psychological Stress and Well-being: A Systematic Review and Meta-analysis." *JAMA Internal Medicine* 174, no. 3 (2014): 357–368.

Hackett, Paul G. *Theos Bernard, the White Lama: Tibet, Yoga, and American Religious Life*. New York: Columbia University Press, 2012.

Harrer, Heinrich. *Seven Years in Tibet*. New York: Tarcher/Putnam, 1953.

Hyde, Jesse. "A Death in the Desert." *Psychology Today*, November 5, 2012.

Krakauer, Jon. *Into the Wild*. New York: Villard Books, 1996.

———. *Under the Banner of Heaven: A Story of Violent Faith*. New York: Doubleday, 2003.

Kramer, Joel, and Diana Alstad. *The Guru Papers: Masks of Authoritarian Power.* Berkeley: Frog Ltd., 1993.

———. *The Passionate Mind Revisited: Expanding Personal and Social Awareness.* Berkeley, CA: North Atlantic Books, 2009.

Krishna, Gopi. *The Awakening of Kundalini.* New York: Dutton, 1975.

Lachman, Gary. *Madame Blavatsky: The Mother of Modern Spirituality.* New York: Tarcher/Penguin, 2012.

Lopez, Donald S., Jr. *Buddhism and Science: A Guide for the Perplexed.* Chicago: University of Chicago Press, 2009.

———. *Prisoners of Shangri-La: Tibetan Buddhism and the West.* Chicago: University of Chicago Press, 1997.

Luhrmann, T. M. *When God Talks Back: Understanding the American Evangelical Relationship with God.* New York: Knopf, 2012.

Miklian, Jason. "Rough Cut." *Foreign Policy,* January 2, 2013.

Monkyi, T. "Interview with Geshe Michael Roach & Christie McNally." InfoBuddhism.com, Easter 2003.

Ng, Beng-Yeong. "Qigong-Induced Mental Disorders: A Review." *Australian & New Zealand Journal of Psychiatry* 33, no. 2 (April 1999): 197–206.

Opler, Morris Edward. *An Apache Life-Way: The Economic, Social, and Religious Institutions of the Chiricahua Indians.* Lincoln: University of Nebraska Press, 1941.

Remski, Matthew. "Psychosis, Stabbing, Secrecy & Death at a Neo-Buddhist University in Arizona." *Elephant Journal,* May 4, 2012.

Rinpoche, Sogyal. *The Tibetan Book of Living and Dying.* San Francisco: HarperOne, 1994.

Roberts, David. *Once They Moved Like the Wind: Cochise, Geronimo, and the Apache Wars.* New York: Touchstone, 1993.

Said, Edward W. *Orientalism.* New York: Random House, 1978.

Satchidananda, Sri Swami, trans. *The Yoga Sutras of Patanjali.* Buckingham, VA: Integral Yoga Publications, 1978.

Sweeney, Edwin R., ed. *Making Peace with Cochise: The 1872 Journal of Captain Joseph Alton Sladen.* Norman: University of Oklahoma Press, 1997.

Thurman, Robert A. F., trans. *The Tibetan Book of the Dead.* New Delhi: HarperCollins, 1998.

Trungpa, Chogyam. *Cutting through Spiritual Materialism.* Boston: Shambhala, 2002.

White, David Gordon. *Sinister Yogis.* Chicago: University of Chicago Press, 2009.

Wilson, Liz. *Charming Cadavers*. Chicago: University of Chicago Press, 1996.

———, ed. *The Living and the Dead: Social Dimensions of Death in South Asian Religions*. Albany: SUNY Press, 2003.

Wright, Lawrence. *Going Clear: Scientology, Hollywood, & the Prison of Belief*. New York: Knopf, 2013.

Diamond Mountain Sources

Diamond Cutter. "Geshe Michael Roach's Sexual Conduct with Students." Geshewatch.blogspot.com, July 7, 2006.

McNally, Christie. "Lama Christie's Talk to Retreatants' Families." Asian Classics Institute, 2010.

———. "A Shift in the Matrix." *Scribd*, April 19, 2012.

———. "Letter to Nina Burleigh." *Rolling Stone,* May 20, 2013.

McNally, Lama Christie. *The Tibetan Book of Meditation*. New York: Doubleday, 2009.

McNally, Lama Christie, and Ian Thorson. *Two As One: A Journey to Yoga*. Tucson: Yoga Studies Institute, 2010.

Roach, Geshe Michael. "Using a Flamethrower to Cut Your Nails." Speech at Friends Meetinghouse, New York City, October 31, 1997.

———. *The Garden: A Parable*. New York: Doubleday, 2000.

———. *How Yoga Works*. Diamond Cutter Press, 2004.

———. "An Open Letter from Geshe Michael Roach." *Elephant Journal,* April 26, 2012.

———. "Answers to Questions from Friends." Unfinished. Prepared for Fernanda Santos, 2012.

———. "Essays to Answer Questions from My Friends." Asian Classics Institute, 2012.

———. *The Karma of Love: 100 Answers for Your Relationship*. Diamond Cutter Press, 2013.

Roach, Geshe Michael, and Christie McNally. *The Essential Yoga Sutra: Ancient Wisdom for Your Yoga*. New York: Doubleday, 2005.

Roach, Geshe Michael, and Lama Christie McNally. *The Diamond Cutter: The Buddha on Managing Your Business and Your Life*. New York: Doubleday, 2000.

———. "The Goddess Code." Asian Classics Institute, September 2, 2005.

———. *The Eastern Path to Heaven: A Guide to Happiness from the Teachings of Jesus in Tibet.* New York: Seabury Books, 2008.

Roach, Geshe Michael, Lama Christie McNally, and Michael Gordon. *Karmic Management: What Goes Around Comes Around in Your Business and Your Life.* New York: Doubleday, 2009.

Veenhof, Douglas. *White Lama: The Life of Tantric Yogi Theos Bernard, Tibet's Lost Emissary to the New World.* New York: Harmony, 2011.